Networks and the Future of Medical Practice

Networks and the Future of Medical Practice

Derek van Amerongen

Integrating Physician, Hospital, and Payor

HEALTH ADMINISTRATION PRESS
CHICAGO, ILLINOIS

02 01 00 99 98   5 4 3 2 1

Library of Congress Cataloging-in-Publication Data
Van Amerongen, Derek.
Networks and the future of medical practice / Derek van Amerongen.
     p.   cm.
   Includes bibliographical references and index.
   1. Medicine—Practice—United States—Forecasting.   2. Integrated
   delivery of health care—United States—Forecasting.   I. Title.
   [DNLM: 1. Delivery of Health Care. Integrated—trends—United
   States.   W 84 AA1 V2n 1998]
   R728.V36   1998
   362.1'0973—dc21
   DNLM/DLC   98-15738
   for Library of Congress   CIP

The paper used in this publication meets the minimum requirements of American National Standard for Information Sciences—Permanence of Paper for Printed Library Materials, ANSI Z39.48–1984. ∞ ™

Health Administration Press
A division of the Foundation
   of the American College of
   Healthcare Executives
One North Franklin Street
Chicago, IL 60606-3491
312/424-2800

To the Van Clan:

Corrie, Greg, Gracie, and, especially, Susan

CONTENTS

FOREWORD

AMERICAN MEDICINE is currently in more turmoil than in any time in memory. There is lots of good news. Mortality rates continue to decline, and spectacular products of science continue to help us reverse disease and disability. But we still have higher rates of mortality than most developed countries, at much higher costs. There is significant inequity in health outcomes in American geographic and racial groups, and the unacceptably high number of uninsured patients continues to grow. Employer and governmental concern about costs has begun to slow the rates of increase, but market forces operating primarily to contain costs have raised significant issues regarding inadequate care, resulting in calls for "patient bills of rights" and other regulatory responses. Thoughtful American statesmen of medicine like George Lundberg caution that the historic "rocking horse" between business and professionalism has tilted toward greed, and a *U.S. News & World Report* headline wonders "How Doctors and Patients Ended Up on Opposite Sides."

Managed care plans are taking the brunt of this criticism, given the incentives for providing less care, and the "shotgun marriages" that are required in many markets to organize physician groups where a history and culture of organized group practice does not exist. It is ironic but understandable that concern about quality of care has been fostered by these developments in ways much more potent than in our fee-for-service environment. Such concerns must be addressed and ways of aligning financial incentives to produce better outcomes in addition to reducing expenditures must be found. It would be very unfortunate if such a reaction undermined the extremely positive aspects of managed care development (e.g., financial incentives that lead to cost control, and the organization of patients into groups large enough so that quality and outcomes can be tracked and population health ensured).

This is where Derek van Amerongen's important contribution comes in. An obstetrician-gynecologist first and physician executive second, he cares deeply about the evolution of American medicine and its challenge to deliver value for American patients. From his graduate studies in medical management and his experience as National Medical Director for Anthem Blue Cross and Blue Shield, he has much to offer on how medicine can be restructured to constrain costs and deliver quality at the same time. His challenge is compelling: "It means putting together a system that adds value to the process. Value has to be a watchword going forward for everyone involved in medical care activities. It is no longer sufficient to provide a benefit; we must demonstrate value."

But this is not a theoretical treatise. What you will find here is state-of-the-art thinking about how the medical care system can be organized into networks of physicians and other providers to produce this value. Van Amerongen argues that "networks have blossomed like flowers after the rain" but there has been scant thought to the nature and implication of these networks. "The flurry of network formation has been a reactionary response, akin to the responses of organized medicine to past change." He analyzes opportunities and strategies for hospital networks and provider-sponsored networks, as well as network strategy for academic health centers. In each case, he presents the pros and cons of alternate arrangements, such as mergers versus alliances for hospital networks, in practical ways that reflect his medical management experience.

The author is a clear advocate for networks organized around pro- viders, and for the role of the physician executives in moving such organizations to the production of value. "Provider-sponsored networks have a built-in advantage in their experience to deliver their service piece that is so sought after by consumers." At the same time, van Amerongen is aware of how challenging it will be for many physicians and physician leaders to acquire the skills and attitudes necessary for them to achieve such a leadership role.

In his final chapter, "Beyond Managed Care," we are reminded that administrative arrangements such as networks are simply a means to an end: "The creation of the network must never be mistaken for the com- pletion of the task." He envisions provider networks in alignment with payors as the critical element in data collection for outcomes measure- ment, which in partnership with employers and public health agencies could take responsibility for the population health of a region.

Such a vision would go a long way toward resolving the crisis of purpose and value that confronts medicine at present. This book should be invaluable to those currently trying to organize such networks and a challenge to others who are developing outcome and value measurement systems for the future.

David A. Kindig, M.D., Ph.D.
University of Wisconsin School of Medicine

INTRODUCTION

"Until recently, people rested content because medicine is in good hands. But the unprecedented growth of medicine, the enormous expansion of personnel and facilities, the investment of billions of dollars have created issues from which society cannot escape merely through its own optimism or through confidence in the high character of medical practitioners."

—Ray Lyman Wilbur, chairman,
Congressional Committee on the Cost of Medical Care, 1933

EVERYTHING YOU know is wrong. This seems to be the message for everyone involved in healthcare today. The motivation for becoming involved is still valid: the desire to provide people with quality medical care. This is the objective, unemotional rationale. But beneath this, we are all dealing with the traditional images of physicians as healers and hospitals as havens. Norman Rockwell paintings and Dr. Kildare movies from the 1940s created this "golden era of medicine" mind-set. The influence of these icons from a vanished time is still strong. Part of the resistance of the medical community to change has been based on a longing for a "reality" that never really existed. A classic doctor joke reflects this: How many physicians does it take to change a light bulb? One—and six to reminisce about how wonderful the old one was.

Medicine has never been a source of cultural change. Through history it has tended to follow or, at best, keep up with changes in society. Some scientists have induced fundamental changes in society. Renaissance astronomers overthrew the entire conception of the universe. Warriors, explorers, and kings forced, pushed, or led societies down paths they might not have otherwise taken. But physicians are by nature conservative. We can accept and even promote innovation within the discipline, but we have not historically been "change leaders." That is why the current upheaval in American healthcare is so painful. It has been thrust upon the healthcare sector by outside forces. People who have never set foot in a hospital are making monumental decisions about health.

Doctors and healthcare executives are still somewhat in shock over how fast this issue has taken center stage. In the mid-1980s, I worked for a staff model health maintenance organization (HMO); no one cared about costs then. The HMO did not even know what it spent on medical care per month. It didn't matter. Year after year, it, and the hospital that owned it, made money—a lot of it.

> Typically we speak of the U.S. "healthcare system." I have a certain reluctance to do so, since our system has done a poor job of creating "health" in this country. We're No. 1 in the world for gross domestic product (GDP) devoted to medical care but our health statistics are dismal. We would be more correct in speaking of the U.S. "medical care" system since we are a long way from developing a true healthcare system. But out of habit and sloth, I will frequently follow convention (or fiction) and use the term "healthcare" in referring to the American medical system.

A Bit of History

How did we get here? A history lesson of sorts is in order. First, we must recognize that only in this century have physicians attained their present vaunted position. Prior to 1900, they were one more class of tradesmen. Only a tiny number practiced in hospitals or even had admitting privileges (Starr 1982). The practice pattern of most doctors was to establish an office at a busy location and stay there. If you were not in your office, potential (paying) patients could not find you. Two technological advances freed the practitioner from being bound to one spot: the telephone and the automobile. It became possible to call ahead and see if the doctor was in. The doctor could call and reschedule patients if needed. Home visits could be accomplished more rapidly, bringing in income and preserving the revenue-generating office hours.

Before World War II, most physicians were general practitioners. "Specialists" were few and far between, and they were centered in big city universities (Starr 1982). Hospitals were generally perceived as places to rest or die. Given the state of medicine at the time, relatively little could be done for most diseases. Most births occurred in the home. Cancer was largely incurable. Most people did not live long enough to develop the diseases of aging. It's not surprising that until the mid-1950s, the most complicated piece of equipment in the hospital was the elevator.

Medical societies, particularly the American Medical Association (AMA), lived in a state of reaction rather than proaction (Garceau 1941). Their main purpose was to preserve the economic status of doctors. This included fighting competing practitioners such as homeopaths and osteopaths and lobbying for exclusivity of the right to practice through licensure. Periodically, usually after great national crises, the subject of national health insurance would come to the fore of political discussion.

We often think of the events of the last five to ten years as the origin of the medical care debate, but its roots are quite deep. Europe, especially Germany, had "sickness plans" in place well before 1900 (Evans 1994). In 1917, during the Depression, and after World War II, attempts were made to pass such legislation in the United States. Each time, organized medicine fought these measures. Interestingly, there was usually little discussion of alternative solutions to the healthcare crises of those times (almost identical to the crises we are dealing with today such as cost, access, incentives for physicians, etc.). Rather, it was the status quo, faults and all, that was so vociferously defended. This is not meant as a slap against organized medicine. It is relevant because it laid the foundation for the approach physicians, and later hospitals, have long taken to healthcare change: resistance, preservation of the status quo, and the development of a "small businessman" mentality around economic issues.

This mind-set went into high gear after World War II. The war had created intense demand for every type of specialist. By the late 1940s, the United States was beginning to see the shift of physicians away from primary care. This shift persists today (Phelps 1992). Most importantly, the business model that American medicine would follow for decades was being formulated. This model was little changed until the late 1980s and is still unchanged in many non-urban areas. In this model, a hospital, the locus of technology in the community, is the delivery site for all acute and most chronic care. Attending physicians treat their patients there and use its services, but are neither employees nor employers in the hospital. Their practices "orbit" the hospital and provide the ambulatory service component. Most physicians who have been in practice (as well as anyone familiar with TV shows from the 1950s and 1960s) will recognize this model immediately. The hospital and the private practice were symbiotic: neither could exist alone. Each complemented the other.

The final piece of the system was the payor. Until the postwar period, this was the individual who was ill. In the 1950s it became the Blue Cross plan or the large employer that offered health insurance of some type. In the 1960s, the government became highly involved through Medicare and Medicaid. But until very recently, the entity footing the bill was regulated to an entirely passive role. The physicians and hospital were handed the "keys to the treasury," as Uwe Reinhardt puts it (Carlson 1997). No questions were asked by any of the participants in the process (patient, doctor, employer, insurer, society), as long as the bills were paid promptly. Meanwhile, the costs of the system rose exponentially.

> "The price of health care services has risen steadily, to a total of $815 billion per year [as of 1996], or 11 percent of the GDP. Health care goods, including medicine, bring the total to 15 percent. If nothing significant is done, the services bill alone will be $2.2 trillion . . . by 2010, when baby boomers start retiring."
> –William Mundell, CEO, WEFA/Primark, 1997

Healthcare Today

We are now well aware of the change that has overwhelmed healthcare since the late 1980s. Managed care seemed to burst on the national scene after years of incubation on the West Coast and a few selected areas in the East. The national healthcare expenditure finally reached a critical mass in 1992, forcing it onto the stage of the presidential campaign debates. For the first time, broad segments of the country became aware of the problems that had up until that point worried only a few health economists. What are we getting for our healthcare dollars (of which there are billions)? How can we improve quality of care? How do we deal with millions of uninsured (whose existence was not even recognized by most)? Is our "medical business model" still valid for the 1990s and beyond?

These are all vital questions. They have led to a tumultuous few years of change. The character of that change has been hotly debated, but there has been little analysis of the kinds of responses that providers—hospitals and physicians—have mounted to deal with this new era. Networks have blossomed like flowers after the rain and, like flowers, there has been scant thought given to the nature and implication of these networks as they pop up almost everywhere. This has led me to focus on network formation and ask some questions. What I have found is that the flurry of network formation has been a *reactionary* response, similar to the previous responses of organized medicine to change. And like those responses to previous crises, the current one has missed the point. Networks have become, in a matter of only two to three years, the stock answer of hospitals and their physician staffs. But simply signing up a list of doctors and holding it out as a functioning entity is not enough to win, and service, a contract. This has been the sad result in communities across

Figure 1.1 The Rise in Uninsured Americans . . .

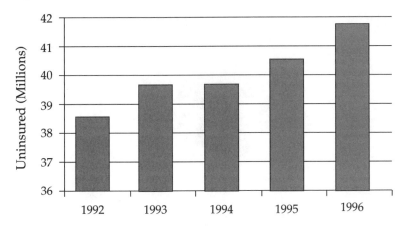

Source: Census Bureau 1997.

the country. Size is not automatically strength. *Smart* network formation means putting together a system that adds value to the process. Value has to be a watchword going forward for everyone involved in medical care activities. It is no longer sufficient to provide a benefit; value must be demonstrated. This will be discussed at length later in the book, but it must be kept in mind from the outset.

There is now a growing problem in medical care decision making of the lack of a "competency imperative." I see a major flaw in the network strategy—as well as much of the strategy that has led to the building of most hospital systems—as being an "all things for all people" approach. But we are moving at breakneck speed into an era of customization and attention to the specific demands of the marketplace. In business, we have seen huge conglomerates sell off the diverse holdings they acquired in the 1970s and 1980s when the mantra was "bigger is better." Now the move is to focus on core business (i.e., core competency). What do physicians do best? What is the real population a hospital is trying to serve? These questions inevitably lead us to concentrate on the competency of the partners in a medical care delivery system, and hopefully will bring us to utilize them most effectively. Any strategy that pulls us away from promoting and fostering the competencies of the various members of the project will not be successful in the long term.

There is a reason that a detailed discussion of networks is particularly appropriate at this time. As we move toward the end of the decade, and managed care accelerates (despite the current backlash of consumer groups and legislators [Kassirer 1997]), every provider must soon make

Figure 1.2 . . . Is but One of the Drivers in the Rise of Managed Care

Employees with Each Type of Coverage: 1993

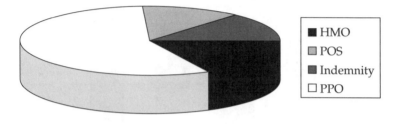

Employees with Each Type of Coverage: 1996

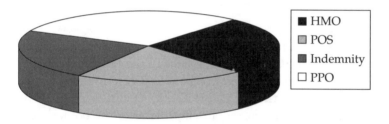

Source: Wm. Mercer, *Wall Street Journal*, October 23, 1997, A3.

the decision of which direction to pursue. Whichever road is chosen will likely commit one to a particular course of action for the next two to five years. By the end of this period, it may well be that the opportunity to move in a different direction, dictated by the pattern of change, is gone and one is left with a losing proposition. Choosing a strategy has never been as important, or as unclear, in medicine as it is today.

Table 1.1 Scope of the Problem: Growth in National Health Expenditures, 1960–90

	1960	1970	1980	1990
Expenditures in Billions Per Capita	$27.1	$74.4	$250.1	$675.0
As % of GDP	5.3	7.4	9.2	12.2
Growth Rate	—	10.6%	12.9%	11.7%

Source: Health Care Financing Administration, Office of the Actuary, 1992.

Table 1.2   What Do We Get for Our Expenditures on Medical Care?

| | Health Outcomes in OECD Countries, 1990 | | |
	Infant Mortality (deaths/1000 live births)	Life Expectancy at Birth (males)	Life Expectancy at Birth (females)
OECD Average	9.7	72.6	78.8
Japan	4.6	75.9	81.9
Finland	5.6	70.9	78.9
Canada	6.8	73.8	80.4
U.K.	7.9	73.0	78.5
Spain	7.8	73.2	80.3
U.S.	9.1	72.0	78.8
Greece	9.7	74.1	78.6

Source: *OECD Health Systems: Facts and Trends.* Paris: Organization for Economic Cooperation and Development, 1993.

How to Use This Book

This book was written for two primary audiences: healthcare executives and physician executives. Healthcare executives have had a long history in medical care delivery with their competent administration of the center of the delivery system for the last 50 years, the hospital. They have since branched out in the newer forms of ancillary services, including the insurance carriers that were once simply passive, claims-paying entities. These executives are now being called on to make assessments of far more than their institution's immediate environment and strategy. Their decisions will sometimes determine whether these facilities live or die.

Physician executives are new to the playing field. In the decades before World War II, most hospitals were led by physicians. They were replaced by professional hospital administrators, the predecessors of healthcare executives. With their retreat from that administrative role, doctors turned their attention to the business of running a private practice. Only in the last ten years have physicians returned in force to the administrative side. This time they are often equipped with advanced training in business and medical administration. Combined with their medical experience, they are uniquely qualified to be at the table in formulating strategy for the future.

Both of these professionals need to understand the trends that are appearing and being reshaped almost daily. It is for these executives that this book is written. It is understood that often the healthcare executive and the physician executive will be in sync in their opinions and strategy. But there will also be divergence on a regular basis, because of their different backgrounds and constituencies. The Venn diagrams of their activities and decisions overlap, but incompletely.

What are the key concepts to draw from the discussions to follow? This book is not meant to be a "how to," with diagrams to cut out and paste in a strategic plan. I hope to provoke thought, encourage exploration down different paths, and enable the reader to feel more prepared to ask and answer critical questions about his or her future directions. A set of key concepts, which are summarized in Table 1.3, will become evident in the chapters to follow. There may be other important lessons beyond the ones listed below that are meaningful based on one's individual setting and circumstances; if so, all the better.

- Focus on core competencies. What is it you do well? Define it, and then seek to make that the strategic focus of your organization.
- Avoid the rush to consolidate as a reaction to change (versus attempting to manage change). Rushing has resulted in physicians and hospitals failing to consider the long-range effects of their decisions and how those decisions fit into new healthcare philosophies, not just how to increase market share in the next quarter.
- Add value. Any new approach to delivering care has to have value as a fundamental attribute (this is really important).
- Bring down traditional boundaries. The old relationships, especially those held at arm's length, do not work anymore. New partnerships must be entertained, even if they are disorienting at first (remember, there would be no Hard Rock Cafe–Beijing or Shanghai Marriott if President Richard Nixon had not gone to China).
- Share education and information liberally, and involve all the potential participants in new ventures: providers, physicians, payors, carriers, patients, employers, etc. This open exchange will then help craft the new system. Do not waste time debating the wisdom of moving forward. "Gain power by accepting reality," as the Chinese proverb says.

The next decade will be the era of population-based medicine. Outcomes, health status, determinants of health—all will be part of the measurements made and analyzed. We cannot do it yet; our systems are still not that sophisticated. But the theory is there and the new structures that will be able to accommodate this view of the world will be superior to those that cannot. In the meantime, it is important to develop this mind-set, since this will speed the entire process.

Remember: *medical care* is not *healthcare*; one delivers care to an individual, the other seeks to raise the health status of an entire community.

"Chance favors the prepared mind."

–Louis Pasteur

We are competent at the former but have a long way to go to achieve the latter.

- Expect to do well economically even as the system continues to evolve. This will not be automatic, but, despite the pressures of managed care, benefits will accrue to those medical groups and providers who innovate, accept, and work with new ideas and tend to "think outside the box." The key is not to let a group be stampeded by a fear of loss of revenue into a poorly conceived project.
- Be committed. Last, but crucial, healthcare executives and physician executives must commit themselves to be the leaders of change. They must be prepared to shoulder their way to the table when critical decisions are discussed and strategy plotted. They must be willing to say the emperor has no clothes and hence, prevent major errors arising from adherence to outdated models. They must acquire and use the skills that will place them in the front rank of their companies' leaders.

If the current trend of network formation is flawed, how did this happen? What does it mean for hospitals? physicians? academic medical centers? What is a viable solution that will permit providers to continue to play a central role? These are the issues we will discuss, as well as attempt to divine the future trends for the new provider combinations that networks represent.

References

Carlson, R. P. 1997. "Health Care Futures: Where Are We Going?" *Physician Executive* 23 (5): 14–26.

Table 1.3 Themes of This Book

- Understand your core competencies and focus on them
- Gain power by accepting reality
- Acknowledge the changing direction of the healthcare delivery system, and determine how to be part of it
- Understand the mechanisms for financial reward in the future
- Understand that success will come to those who improve healthcare delivery and achieve better outcomes

Evans, R. G. 1994. *Why Are Some People Healthy and Others Not?* New York: Aldine de Gruytor.

Garceau, O. 1941. *The Political Life of the American Medical Association.* Boston: Harvard University Press.

Kassirer, J. P. 1997. "Practicing Medicine Without a License: The New Intrusions by Congress." *New England Journal of Medicine* 336: 1747.

Phelps, C. E. 1992. *Health Economics.* New York: HarperCollins.

Starr, P. 1982. *The Social Transformation of American Medicine.* New York: Harper Collins.

2

HOSPITAL-SPONSORED NETWORKS

"The hospital sees its assets like old children's clothes: they still fit, so their answer is to have more children."

—Thomas Royer, M.D., chairman,
board of governors, Henry Ford Health System, 1993

HOSPITALS ARE unlike any other industry. This seems obvious, and it is, but not necessarily for the reasons most think. Prior to 1945, hospitals were almost social institutions. Without antibiotics, sophisticated equipment, or much medical knowledge, care consisted of providing a community of dedicated workers to support the patient's own healing process. This "caring mission" became the heart of the hospital's compact with patients and the community at large. In 1938, when the average daily cost of a hospital bed was $4, it was a very good deal for all involved. By 1969, *Life* magazine featured advertisements asking "With hospital costs at $54 a day, how lucky will you be?" (1969). Such prices look ludicrous to us today. But it highlights the fundamental shift in the way medicine has been delivered in the United States.

Over the last 20 years, we have experienced a dramatic role reversal in how medical delivery is performed. Traditional fee-for-service is individual-based and measured (if at all) by short-term outcomes (did the patient leave the operating room alive). It has been centered on the inpatient experience. Managed care has up-ended this equation. Population-based treatments, long-term outcomes (what is the patient's functioning at 6 and 12 months after surgery; when will the patient be able to resume normal activity, including a return to work), and a longitudinal view of the care process are all part of the "paradigm shift" brought by managed care. The inpatient experience becomes only one of several modules of care (ambulatory, outpatient, home care, etc.). These changes are problematic for hospitals for a variety of reasons. The solution many have selected is to form a network. The trend toward forming networks stems from several areas of trouble that have recently beset the modern hospital.

Hospitals have come to be seen as the hub of the local medical community around which the physicians array their practices. The recent trend toward "hospitalists" (Wachter 1996) may well free many doctors from needing hospital privileges, but *that is still in the future*. In a larger sense, the community hospitals then "orbit" around the local or regional academic medical centers for tertiary care. The unique issues of academic medical centers will be explored later. But as new patterns of care gain momentum, these hub-and-spoke arrangements are being disrupted.

Private physicians have never been employees of hospitals but have always occupied a sort of netherworld unduplicated in any other profession; they are *in* the institution but not *of* it. A landmark legal case from 1957, *Darling v. Charleston Community Memorial Hospital*, established the responsibility of the hospital to oversee the physicians who work there but left intact their independence (Furrow 1991). It also preserved the ability to generate revenue within the walls of the hospital without having to share that revenue. Until recently, this holding has been a plus for hospitals. They could entice physicians onto their staffs and obtain a piece of their inpatient pie. They could maintain an arm's-length relationship with the doctors and insulate themselves from practice issues that arise outside of the inpatient setting. Now, however, these positives have all turned sour. The physicians' divided loyalties make them easier prey for managed care organizations (MCOs) and other hospitals that have begun to request a certain amount of exclusivity.

Without a financial arrangement, the only leverage many hospitals have with their medical staffs is friendly persuasion. Against dollars, it is not a very effective tool. The rise in the status of the primary care physician (PCP) is also troubling. Hospitals tend to be overloaded with specialists. The few physicians employed by hospitals have usually been specialists (anesthesiologists, radiologists, pathologists, etc.), none of whom directly generate patient flow or revenue. Hence hospitals have been pressed to find a means to bring on more PCPs because that is what (they think) MCOs and the government want. This is a daunting task considering the PCP "shortage" (Christianson et al. 1995). Many nonrural hospitals have ratios of 3 or 6 to 1 (specialty care physician [SCP] to PCP). As late as 1997, the Johns Hopkins Hospital in Baltimore, with more than 1,000 beds and close to 1,500 physicians on staff, had fewer than five family physicians with admitting privileges, and its School of Medicine had no Department of Family Practice.

Hospitals also tend to have their own vision of their role and value to the community. Study after study shows we are significantly overbedded in all parts of the United States (*Modern Healthcare* 1995c; *Cincinnati Enquirer* 1997). Many other industries have eliminated this overcapacity in order to render the U.S. economy more efficient to compete globally (*New York Times* 1997). But the special character of hospitals as a "community asset" (i.e., a facility that is of value to the community for various reasons, including economically, medically, socially) prevents this trend from being replicated. For example, a hospital in Florida that wished to merge with another just a couple of miles away would have eliminated about half of the total beds between the two at a time when occupancy for both was less than 60 percent. The move was blocked by the board of trustees who represented local businessmen, physicians, and community activists. They stopped the merger on the grounds that it would remove an important local asset (*Modern Healthcare* 1997a). While it was true the hospital had long been a source of community pride, a provider of jobs, and a place to do volunteer work, it was also usually operating at a loss. Meanwhile, an equally satisfactory facility, also underutilized, was only minutes away. In any other kind of business, the economic imperatives would have clearly led to consolidation and resulting efficiencies for the entire community. Yet due to an activist board (and probably a few "Casino Night" fund raisers, an option unavailable to a truly competitive business), the money-losing facility is still in operation. It should be noted that the healthcare executives involved understood the validity of consolidation but were frustrated by the board structure, which prevented the hospitals from becoming more efficient.

The communications revolution has put us well on the way to a "virtual society." More and more businesses function on the Internet and with reduced overhead, especially in the service sector. Hospitals, meanwhile, continue to have huge assets tied up in bricks and mortar. In more than 20 years in medicine, I have never been in a hospital that was not undergoing some sort of renovation or construction. Constant growth has been the mantra of hospital executives, fueled in part by the favorable treatment of such activity by Medicare (Phelps 1992). It is a visible legacy for an administration or board to leave behind and proof to the community of the hospital's engagement. But it is no longer supportable. MCOs do not want to pay for it, and Medicare and the states are restructuring to remove the incentives (*Wall Street Journal* 1997a). What to do then with these buildings that represent so much time, effort, and other people's money (and often their names as well)?

Academic medical centers (AMCs) have additional problems. First, their facilities are usually even larger than any other hospital in town. Aside from the support functions needed for a larger number of beds, those beds tend to be of higher acuity and require more ancillary services. Add to this the research and teaching missions, and the square footage becomes immense. AMCs are also frequently one of the largest employers in the area. Thus, any restructuring runs up against labor unions, local economic forces, and even local ordinances and regulations. Universities may devote disproportionate segments of their budgets to the academic medical activities. According to the Budget Report of the American Association of Medical Colleges, two or three hundred medical students may "eat up" two-thirds of the operating budget of a 15,000-student university (1995).

Finally, this is an era when employers have reached unparalleled levels of sophistication in healthcare evaluation and purchasing (General Electric 1997). The products offered by an insurer have therefore become increasingly important in predicting patient flow. The breadth of options available to a member determines more than ever whether an institution will be able to capture business, hence revenue. As MCOs develop new and innovative products to meet the shifting demands of employers, fewer revolve around the hospital. More MCOs tend toward the ambulatory encounter as the focal point, using such things as multidisciplinary panels, etc. (*Managed Healthcare* 1997). This leaves the hospitals out in the cold, a major change from the insurance plans of just a few years ago. Hospitals have had to scramble to still be seen as players.

In summary, hospitals entered the '90s with substantial baggage, not the least of which was their fragmented organizational response to managed care (*Managed Healthcare* 1997). Some would designate one or more individuals in the hospital administrative structure as "responsible" for managed care development. This person would then seek to contract with the various MCOs, often with no experience or training in managed care issues. Even as disjointed as this approach is, it still far outstrips the efforts the physician community has been able to mount on any kind of broad scale. For with all their burdens, hospitals still possess three advantages in the medical marketplace:

1. They are not physicians and so are not as bound as many doctors are by the ostrich-like response to change.
2. They are businesses, for all their insulation from true competition and real-world economic forces. They have an infrastructure of sorts and some experience and familiarity with the requirements of running a large enterprise.
3. They are repositories of a fair amount of capital.

Hospitals were thus positioned to step into the vacuum that appeared when physicians failed to initially present a coordinated plan to deal with managed care and the new power that employers and insurers were exerting. The requests of employers fell, as a result, on deaf ears in organized medicine. Those requests included more coordination of care, more PCPs, reductions in the cost of care, outcomes reporting, and accountability. With their "corner grocer" style of business, most small group practices were in no state to even consider meeting these challenges. Indeed, the vast majority of physicians had no idea what these concepts meant. It is certainly questionable how many physicians have addressed this knowledge deficit in the last four to six years. Of course, hospital executives did not necessarily understand them either. The business purpose of their facilities, involving as it did (and still does) maximizing cash flow while maintaining overcapacity, is in direct conflict with the philosophy of managed care. But being the only organized medical unit on the block with some business savvy, not to mention money, hospitals were uniquely positioned to step into the breach.

The Development of Hospital-Sponsored Networks

The answer to that problem was to gain control of the sources of patient flow. (A Marxist, if one still existed, would say the hospitals wanted to control the means of production!) This would entail somehow locking in the staff physicians and directing their admissions and other services to the hospital. If possible, it would also mean boosting the volumes of those services. This poses an interesting dilemma for hospitals that have always claimed an arm's length relationship to the physicians who walk the halls but are "voluntary" staff.

Yet it was obvious that the business model in place since the 1950s was in turmoil. Time—usually seen as a benefit to medicine because it has inevitably brought more innovation, more technology, and large profit margins—has become an enemy. With the failure of President Clinton's health reform plan, the locus of the reform movement was firmly situated in the private sector. The government would continue to significantly influence medical care because of the huge budgets of the Health Care Financing Administration (HCFA) and the Department of Defense, but the initiative would now be with the market forces. There was no longer the luxury of waiting to see how changes in healthcare would resolve themselves. No one could sit by the sidelines. Everyone had to choose a direction and create a strategy eventually. Waiting meant that by the time trends became absolutely clear, it might well be too late to take full advantage of that knowledge. Hospitals were thrust into the role of declaring a course of action with only partial information. Given that most hospitals were, and are, managed by administrators raised in the indemnity world of fee-for-service reimbursement, this is a leap. To choose unwisely may have severe negative repercussions, but to *fail* to choose at all could be fatal.

It is important to understand this state of mind to put into context the rise of hospital-sponsored networks (HSNs). I have chosen this term instead of the more common physician-hospital organization (PHO) for several reasons. First, "PHO" implies that physicians have had a leading role in the formation of PHOs. This is rarely so, as will be made plain when we discuss the characteristics of an HSN. Physicians are certainly key, but in general they are not the motivators and have been lackluster partners with the hospitals for a variety of reasons. "PHO" also suggests that there is some equality between the two groups, which is also false. "HSN" is a more descriptive and accurate term.

HSNs are highly reactive. They are designed to fill a void and to do it fast. They have often been organized without a clear view as to their role in the long-term future of medical care delivery or what they mean to the process of integrating care. Nevertheless, they represent an important natural development in the evolution of delivery systems. Despite the lack of groundwork preceding them and the uncertainty of their roles, they have become an omnipresent feature on the medical landscape. The basic issue for everyone interested in health economics, especially physicians, is what utility HSNs may ultimately bring to the practice of medicine.

HSNs have certain characteristics that define, as well as limit, them:

- They are hospital initiated, with physicians as partners but not necessarily equal ones. Their governance and structure are established by the hospital, with varying input from the doctors. Often, such input is minimal. This reflects the generally passive role most physicians have taken throughout most of the healthcare debate. It is a stance that has not exactly covered the physician community with glory. We can be extremely vocal in opposition to another agency's actions, but we rarely act in a proactive manner. As a consequence, a gap has existed that the hospitals have understandably moved to fill. It also illustrates why the term "PHO" is a misnomer.

- They are funded and capitalized by the hospitals. The theory is that once the network becomes a going concern, with a certain volume of patients, it will become self-sufficient. Note that this critical mass consists of patients, not physicians. It is easy to staple together a large number of doctors without having that translate into meaningful patient flow. I have worked with health plans in California (a particularly physician-rich environment) where the doctor to member ratio can easily be 100 to 1. Regardless, many nascent HSNs will go on record as predicting self-sufficiency within one to three years (Clay 1995b). (It is possible to do your own impromptu test of the truth of this statement by contacting the PHO at your hospital and asking about their cash-flow situation. It has now been one to three years for many of them and we should have seen this financial independence come to pass.)

- There is a stated acknowledgment by the hospitals that the purpose of the network is *not* to fill beds. At issue is whether this is a true realization of the hospital and whether they appreciate that under managed care many beds will not only be unfilled, but will have to be eliminated. For hospital systems, composed of several individual facilities, this becomes even more difficult. How does one choose which one will bear the brunt of the reduction in overcapacity?

- The network is seen by the sponsor as a means of rapid entry into a managed care market. As previously mentioned, time is of the essence. The fear is not only of losing one's staff to another institution, but also the threat of market entry of new competitors who are better prepared and more experienced. A network becomes a shortcut to that end.

- There may or may not be an associated insurance product. This definitely requires a fair degree of sophistication and capital. The examples where it has been successful are few. This characteristic will be dealt with in a later section. Suffice it to say that the lure of adding a product to complement the delivery system is strong, but it is a treacherous path.

- A prime objective is to prepare physicians to accept and manage risk. In some regards, the HSN almost becomes an in vivo experiment that the hospital hopes will lay the foundation for accepting capitation. As Medicare risk contracting spreads and hospitals expand into long-term care and home care, this will take on added importance.

- The network is designed to act as a negotiating agent for contracts for the participating physicians and their practices. Hospitals have perceived this as desirable to MCOs: single signature authority to bind doctor and hospital, ambulatory and inpatient modules. The question is whether that single signature can later be translated into action at the point of service. (van Amerongen 1997)

This picture of HSNs will be useful in the discussions to follow. One caveat: certainly many examples of hospital-sponsored entities can be found that do not fit this mold precisely. The same can be said for any attempt to define a highly idiosyncratic organizational framework. But it is a solid start and will allow us to compare apples to apples.

How to Define Success

The formation of a network is a means to an end. This simple fact is frequently forgotten in the rush to consolidate medical organizations and providers. What does "success" mean? Surprisingly, I have often found confusion on the part of network executives when this question is raised. Referring back to our list, the "stated" objective is not to fill beds, but this can easily become the unspoken goal. A second misconception is to relate success to entirely economic indicators. In this way of thinking, any network that can show a surplus (even if this "profit" is derived from interest income), or at least be on budget (since it is likely most start-up projects will have a negative cash flow for the initial period), is successful. This interpretation misses the point. To be successful, a network should do three things.

1. Affect the bottom lines of the participating providers in a meaningful way

This success factor can apply to HSNs, physician-sponsored networks (PSNs), and other networks. The most important word here is "meaningful." Until the hospital or group sees the network as significantly affecting the profit and loss statement, there will be little motivation to provide anything more than lip service to the objectives of integrating to deliver better care. To paraphrase Lyndon Johnson, "when you have them by the wallets, their hearts and minds will follow." As much as organized medicine, especially the AMA, hates capitation, health plans turned to it almost out of desperation in order to get the providers' attention and make them take the managed care principles seriously. Likewise, the financial benefits of participating in and supporting the network must be real and easily identifiable for the provider members.

2. Provide a rationale for participating physicians to prefer the network over other options

This goes to the heart of what it means to bring people together in a collaborative effort. Part of the thesis of this book is that the stampede to consolidate and align has prevented hospitals and doctors from carefully considering the long-range effects of their decisions. Each hospital sees its network as unique, just as it feels its mission is unique among all other hospitals in town. Yet the practitioner sees these HSNs as merely variations on a theme, and not necessarily a very exciting one. The doctor has become used to dealing with a dozen or more different insurers, all of whom are more alike than different. The various networks are similar. The problem then is how to persuade the doctor, a participant in multiple networks, to use one over another, bringing along patients and revenue, thereby increasing the chance of achieving the first success factor. Therein lies the rub.

This also involves providing value back to the physician. This "value exchange" must be multidirectional. A network must structure itself so physicians become more competitive as a result of participating (Callahan et al. 1995). For example, reduction of administrative overhead and red tape can be a lure to participation (*Medical Herald* 1995), as is single signature contracting mentioned in the list above. The concept of value delivered to the physician is a major topic of Chapter 3.

3. Lay the groundwork for future relationships

This element is almost always overlooked. While the pace of change seems to be breakneck, to some observers it is only beginning to accelerate.

> "I view the war on health care costs and the quality issue as [thus far] basically some skirmishes on the fringes . . . They took out a few machine gun nests, but . . . the pillboxes are still there, fully manned. I predict a second major war is going to come."
>
> –Uwe Reinhardt, Ph.D., Princeton University (Inglehart 1997)

Networks can provide a singularly useful service to their hospital and physician members by preparing them for the next stages of medical care delivery evolution. None of us should be confused into thinking that what we call "managed care" is the endpoint of the change process. No doubt we will look back someday and be amused at how crude and rudimentary our efforts were, just as when we contrast the hospital of 1920 with that of today. Indeed, with the lightning speed of change, it is probably absurd for us to believe any of the networks that exist now will be long-term players. But the participants can be ready for the next shift in direction for medicine, even as consolidation of the system as a whole continues (Kassirer 1996).

Choosing a Course: Several Caveats

More than ever, hospitals are paying attention to the physicians who walk their halls. The relationship has always been loose, with doctors demanding and receiving a level of autonomy unknown in other professions. The hospitals, of course, have greatly benefited from this scenario, reaping the profits of the billable services ordered by the attendings. As one healthcare executive once asked an assembled group: What is the most expensive piece of equipment in the hospital? It is the doctor's pen, used to order all those tests and procedures. Most leaders in the medical industry have come to see networks—linking the physicians with another entity—as the cornerstone of any successful medical enterprise going forward (Clay 1995a). The short-term view is that this is a way to present themselves to payors in a more attractive format. This presumes that payors (including insurers, employers, and the government) have become the drivers of change. The long-term view is that hospitals see this as a path to accomplishing multiple tasks, of which winning managed care contracts is only one. These tasks include increasing efficiency, downsizing, lowering overhead on remaining services and functions, and generally integrating as well as creating services (Greene 1997).

The golden key is the template that will allow all of this to happen. Selecting this template involves understanding several factors:

- the dynamics and internal politics of the institution;
- the characteristics of the marketplace;
- the status and involvement (or lack thereof) of the medical staff in hospital decision making;
- knowledge of what the hospital *really* wants to accomplish (refer back to the definition of HSNs and the factors for success);
- an appreciation of the timeline this decision will impose on the parties; and
- capital.

The real risk of this process is that we are still in the embryonic stage of managed care. Reinhardt warns us the greatest struggle is yet to come. After all the trauma endured by the medical community over the past few years, this is not easy to hear. Also, networks themselves are impermanent but exist to serve as a necessary evolutionary stage. Any choice will commit an organization to one strategy or another. Hopefully, we will be able to see far enough down the road to avoid some of the potholes.

Patterns of HSN Development

Two basic choices exist for a hospital that wishes to form a viable business venture with providers and/or other hospitals. In a merger, organizations combine to form a new, single entity (Duncan 1995). An alliance is a loosely coupled arrangement among existing organizations designed to achieve some long-term strategic purpose not possible by any one of them alone (Duncan 1995). Each choice has its own pluses and minuses, and each has a role in a given circumstance.

Merger

A merger (or "mi casa es su casa") theoretically leads to the highest level of control, as there is one board or administrative group developing policy. There should follow from this control the ability to accomplish such management goals as allocation of resources in a logical fashion across the merged system. The single philosophy of the unified directors or trustees should avoid the fractional and parochial infighting between member institutions that can arise in looser configurations.

On the medical side, there is great value in the merger concept because it should foster a continuum of care as separate facilities come together and apportion their services in a planned, consistent, comprehensive manner. Patients and physicians would ideally flow seamlessly from one site to another. Medical needs, not turf, would dictate the proper patterns of care. (Doesn't this sound a lot like managed care?) This coordination has an almost irresistible appeal to those healthcare and physician executives who have been frustrated over the difficulty of bringing logical combinations (from a medical delivery viewpoint) together.

I use the terms "theoretically" and "ideally" in describing the merger model simply because it *is* an ideal. Mergers in healthcare have accelerated dramatically in recent years (*Modern Healthcare* 1995b). But healthcare is unlike any other industry. Merger means commingling of assets, with a single bottom line. It means shedding unproductive units and eliminating waste and redundancy. It runs smack up against the entrenched professional boundaries medicine has spent 80 years building. It is one thing for General Motors to close a plant and shift production (not that this is ever easy or free from much pain and effort). It is, however, quite another thing to tell a group of highly trained, highly paid, and highly regarded physicians that their department will no longer be needed.

For the healthcare systems willing to bite this very large bullet, there can be some major rewards. The Catholic hospital systems have done perhaps more consolidating than others because of their similarities of mission and religious linkages. The St. Francis Healthcare System in Cincinnati laid out several clearly focused objectives in its merger with several other Franciscan hospitals:

- greater efficiency in delivery of healthcare services;
- reduction in duplication of services;
- improved geographic dispersion;

- increased service scope;
- restraint in price increases; and
- improved financial performance. (Roggy and Gorrity 1993)

Note that these are interrelated and mutually reinforcing objectives. They would help any organization truly integrate the functions that both deliver care and support that delivery model. This is the powerful attraction of the merger approach. It meshes nicely with the long-term goal of becoming a managed care player.

Role of Physicians

None of these advantages comes without a price. Consider that merger means generating a single financial structure, a single way of operating, and a new identity. Such a fundamental transformation of an organism as inherently conservative as a hospital is not without serious disadvantages. It is hardly a given that a unified board would be able to exert its authority and accomplish the endpoint of a single strategy across the company. The control it has may well be illusory. Physicians in various settings may or may not subscribe to the newly merged corporation's goals. Even mergers involving millions of dollars and thousands of employees can be torn asunder over such issues. This resistance may be overt, covert, or passive. It may emanate from a department that does not even directly generate patient revenue or seem to be a political base. It is important that the planners of such initiatives remember that any change that could be interpreted as limiting physician autonomy has potential for conflict, which could consume the entire process.

Solutions to this conflict involve generating support among the medical staff. The first step is education and information-sharing. This must be done from day one and in as open a manner as possible. It is fascinating to see multi-million dollar deals set in motion without any consideration of the wishes of the physicians who would be intimately

A rather dramatic example of the collapse of an attempted merger occurred in New York in early 1997. Mt. Sinai and New York University sought to merge their hospitals and medical schools, in part a result of managed care and declining reimbursements and in part to complement each other's strengths. After several years and millions of dollars in preliminary work, the proposed marriage collapsed over cultural issues such as who would be the chair of a consolidated department and where the medical students would take certain classes (*Wall Street Journal* 1997c). These were not simply turf or ego problems, but basic conflicts between two large institutions with very different traditions.

affected, and who are the principal sources of revenue. A survey done of the CEOs of several large urban hospitals that planned to merge showed that only one bothered to include the physician representatives at the start of the talks (van Amerongen 1996). Two of the hospitals actually allowed the deliberations to proceed to the stage of being announced to the press before informing their physicians.

Why does this happen? Many possible explanations exist. The typical healthcare executive may see the doctors as disinterested parties, who only come to the hospital to walk the wards and then leave. This was certainly valid in the past, but the recent upheaval in medicine has served to focus doctors as never before on these nonclinical medical issues. Their interest level is at an all-time high. There is also a lack of appreciation for the autonomy concerns of physicians, which may be another reason for excluding physicians from merger discussions. There is a suspicion that the physicians really don't care and would rather ignore the business aspects of the hospital's affairs. This can lead to a questioning of the loyalty of the physician staff to the hospital and the sense that this limited commitment does not justify bringing the medical staff into these discussions at an early stage.

Some or all of these assumptions may be correct in any particular situation at any given time. But it is necessary for the hospital executive staff to reexamine its approach to physician involvement in these strategic processes if the buy-in is going to be there. Otherwise, one has a recipe for failure. Regardless of the track record of physicians, which has been lackluster, this is a new scenario. The decisions concerning network development reach far beyond the hospital campus and into the very practices of the physicians who work there. Even if past involvement in hospital operations, including support for needed changes, has been minimal, the advent of managed care has made physicians more sensitive than ever to how their environment is structured.

There is another downside to not bringing the physicians along from the start of any major project. By freezing them out (either purposely or not), the opportunity to nurture and train physician leaders as *physician executives* is lost. Future success of hospital systems will depend increasingly on physician executives who are involved, insightful, and inventive. These skills can be acquired only through experience. It then becomes an obligation of the hospital to take responsibility for helping physicians obtain such a background.

From the outset, the leaders of the medical staff must be full partners at the table at the same time full disclosure of the relevant issues and education of the staff regarding new trends and initiatives occur. This is an ideal chance to bring the medical piece into the decision loop. It will help guarantee the project does not proceed without keeping itself grounded in the mission of the institution. This is one of the times when a clear, concise mission statement bears directly on the strategy formulation of the organization; it illustrates why it is so important to have one. I firmly believe that as networks proliferate, and as employers and payors grow more sophisticated, a vital differentiating factor will be the role of physician input to the system. As more large companies take on full-time medical directors to provide medical analysis, they will be looking for the same from the groups with which they contract. This physician role must be a real one. Window dressing is a red flag to well-informed payors. The era of the retired chief of surgery, plaid pants and all, functioning as vice president for medical affairs (at least until he moves to Florida) is, or should be, over. One close look at the structure and functionality of the networks will be enough to make this evident to an astute employer or insurer. This then becomes, like most topics, both a threat and also a tremendous opportunity. The visionary hospital/network leadership that seeks out a similarly visionary physician executive will have a competitive edge. And most important, lest we forget the purpose behind all of this activity, the network will deliver better care.

Local Issues

Having a merged entity does not make local issues disappear. By "local issues" I mean the type of problems that stopped the New York academic centers from merging. Each hospital sees itself as having a unique position in the community. For those with a long history, a religious affiliation or an ethnic one, this is even more true. This "pride of ownership" on the part of special segments of the community has kept more than one hospital in business long after financial events and demographic changes should have closed it (*Wall Street Journal* 1997b). This ability to ignore economic reality has served to isolate the hospital industry as a whole from the same pressures that affect any other business (Phelps 1992).

Clearly many mergers are predicated on the idea that redundant services will be eliminated. As the CEO of a five-hospital system once said, "I don't need five laundries." That is certainly true, and elimination of duplicative support services is an appropriate place to start. This represents, however, the "low-hanging fruit." Once laundry, food, maintenance, delivery, and other services are combined or streamlined, then the hard work begins. The next logical step would be to eliminate redundant clinical services or ones that are poorly utilized or badly managed. This may well mean treading on cherished local programs. These can represent the vested interests of the individual hospitals. Each may have a board of trustees that is reticent to see its obstetrics unit or rehab center be closed in preference to that of a sister hospital. Of the five hospitals in the example mentioned above, the laundries may well have been trimmed, but in year 3 of the merger, not a single bed had been closed (this despite the significant overlap of service areas of the hospitals). Obviously, the concept of increased control arising from the merger model is not easily implemented. This does not make it a less worthy goal to pursue, but it is important to understand that it does not automatically flow from the top down.

Forging a Culture

The operational aspects outlined in bullets above are practical and necessary. Important too is the cultural side of the merger. The organization's ability to blend different values and styles harmoniously has been alluded to but bears additional emphasis. Culture is key: it is how people work and play together. It can be a strong force for binding them or for tearing them apart. The most effective way to deal with both physician and local issues is to forge a new culture. This is a lesson well known in industry. It has often led to the crash and burn of a promising business relationship, not unlike the NYU-Mt. Sinai episode (*Wall Street Journal* 1995). In medicine, we frequently discount such "touchy-feely" ideas as being less important because of the "scientific" nature of what we do. But historically there has been far more art than science in medical practice, especially in the mechanics of medical delivery. Here are several features worth remembering:

- Just as a detailed financial, operational, and structural analysis of the merger partners is done prior to completing the deal (i.e., due diligence), the cultures of the institutions need to be rigorously assessed as well. It is obvious in retrospect why some deals fail: one side did not appreciate the core beliefs of the other; one could not compromise on a given subject important to the other; etc. Culture can also be a means to cement a partnership, as has occurred with several Catholic mergers that trade on the shared traditions of their religious backgrounds.
- Leadership on cultural issues must be crystal clear. There should be no confusion on the part of the staffs as to where the leaders stand. There cannot be a feeling that a hidden reservation exists between the leaders of the soon-to-be-merged organizations.
- Trade on differences when they can be useful and positive. It may be that the organizational behavior of two hospitals is different for a reason, such as significantly different service areas or clientele. With a shared mission and vision uniting them, one can still foster

a certain individuality of each that will assist them in their unique roles.

It is important to understand that creating a unifying culture is an essential part of the merger process. If the goal is simply to bring some hospitals (or any kind of organization, since this concept applies equally to medical groups, plans, etc.) together to save money on uniforms, it will not realize much success. Such a merger does nothing to create a distinctive provider able to differentiate itself in the market and render a unique service. Differentiating oneself can only be done by coupling that economy of scale with a cohesive strategy for the merged group. This strategy must rest on solid values, shared by all and supported by a need on the part of the customer.

It may take several years for the new culture to emerge. This time frame will be hastened if the elements for success mentioned above are present and if a consistent message is broadcast. This message must be a positive one: the trauma of a merger must be put into the context of a necessary evolutionary phase in order to permit the hospital, and the groups that use it, to give better care, which will only be accomplished through its new structure. Generally, this is an understandable message and one that can be made fairly easily if the merger is based on meaningful, shared values and stands for something more than a cheaper way to do business. Since a huge amount of effort, time, money, and moral suasion are essential to make a merger happen, it is not something a farsighted leadership will undertake without a strong personal commitment.

Alliance

Many systems opt for the siren call of alliance (or "merger-lite"). It is in many ways a more efficient route than a merger, but the question that will take some years to answer is whether it will be more effective. Strategic alliances are loosely coupled arrangements between existing organizations designed to achieve some long-term strategic purpose not possible by any individual (Duncan 1995). In a typical alliance, each member purchases an ownership share in the new entity and is represented on the board. A hospital thus retains its autonomy and has the power to sever the relationship if it becomes dissatisfied (Gray 1991). This agreement provides a measure of reassurance to the hospital that it has an escape clause should the arrangement fail to perform as promised, if the institution finds its goals in conflict, if the external environment changes, etc. In theory, the result is a strengthening of the competitive position of each participant while preserving maximum independence.

Alliances thus go beyond normal company-to-company dealings but fall short of being a merger or full partnership. This status underlines the attractiveness of an alliance for all involved. A summary of the principal benefits can be found in Table 2.1. In short, the alliance route is fast and cheap (when compared to a merger) and preserves almost full freedom of action for the members. These benefits may also accrue relatively quickly (more "low-hanging fruit"), giving a boost to the cooperative agreement early in its life. These benefits can act as solutions to a number of competitive and strategic problems hospitals face as they find themselves pressured by the forces of consolidation from the marketplace and increased penetration by managed care.

But these short-term solutions also lay the basis for many of the drawbacks of the alliance option. A careful review of Table 2.1 would show that each of these positives can also lead to significant negatives. The ability to walk away on short notice, perhaps for reasons that have little to do with the alliance itself, means the viability of the new network is always somewhat in doubt. This is a message payors will consider when awarding contracts. Payors are well aware of the maxim that it is one thing to win a contract but another to be able to service it. In a competitive market, where differentiation and focal segmentation are ever more important, any sense of impermanence could scuttle a network's ability to secure contracts. This in turn prevents the critical flow of patients, revenue, and service volume that are necessary to give the network life. Without legal and financial binds joining the hospitals together, there needs to be some mechanism for maintaining the alliance structure short of proceeding to merger. This link may well be an enthusiastic leadership, demonstrating commitment to the project at the local level and involving various stakeholders along the way. A dynamic executive, especially a physician, can be the necessary ingredient to keeping the members allied

Table 2.1   Benefits of the Alliance Model

- New markets can be entered quickly.
- Cultures do not have to be melded.
- Each institution maintains its own bottom line.
- Prized clinical programs can be preserved.
- Autonomy of the various medical staffs is not threatened.
- There is potential to cut costs by reducing some redundant services.
- Financial commitment is usually modest.
- Marketing opportunities exist under the new logo or brand name.
- Independence is maintained to pursue other business opportunities.
- There is an ability to walk away if dissatisfied.

long enough to see the patients begin to roll in (*Modern Healthcare* 1997f).

Alliances facilitate rapid entry into a market. This fact is important when the managed care penetration in an area starts to increase rapidly. Hospitals that have previously been independent suddenly see networks and mergers appearing around them, and panic is just a few deep breaths away. The alliance model can be a quick way of getting into the game, but the alliance must be able to show some sort of plus (as compared to being in the network) in delivery of services and use of resources. The systems that tightly control these elements are already at a distinct advantage (*Modern Healthcare* 1995a). Inability to coordinate care between member hospitals, physician groups, and outpatient services may further hamper an alliance's competitive stature. After all, it is this issue of coordination of care that MCOs are trying to find. They will have little empathy with an alliance partner who insists on maintaining what the MCO considers as redundant services (for example, two open-heart units in a limited service area) and then passing the costs on to the MCO. It is not sufficient simply to consolidate support or ancillary services. While resulting in cost savings, these are not major chunks of the medical care dollar. Their elimination does nothing to attack the core problems of overcapacity and excess utilization of clinical services. It also does not address a cornerstone of managed care philosophy, namely modifying physician behavior to improve outcomes and expand accountability.

This is a daunting task for the alliance. It reiterates the need for strong physician leadership (not just representation) at the very top of the organization. If the individual medical staffs perceive the alliance as mere background noise, it will be completely unable to perform the type of medical management that MCOs and large employers demand. If the alliance is going to function as a sort of Voluntary Hospital Association, it perhaps should not bother. (The Voluntary Hospital Association was created to act as a group purchaser for hospitals to obtain better discounts on supplies and services. It is trying to become a managed care player and provide some managed care support for its members. In most areas, however, its traditional role continues.) MCOs are astute enough to realize this. The burden of proof then shifts to the fledgling alliance, especially if it has yet to handle any significant clinical volume and so has not produced a track record for review. It must be demonstrated that the systems and the political will exist to make the alliance happen at the local level.

The history of merged and allied networks is very brief. A survey by the University of Minnesota Health Research Center showed 70 percent were three years old or less (1996). It may well be that the supposed advantages of merger—control, a single bottom line, elimination of duplicative services, etc.—may never be realized for most merged entities. The main threat to both types of systems is the inability to deliver on contractual obligations. Secondary threats are the failure to get the physicians on board and to convince customers the network is serious about doing business. Issues of infrastructure, shared expertise between members, potential economies of scale, etc., actually are positive for both models. A strong, coordinated alliance can also lead to results compatible to a merger.

How, Then, to Choose?

The trick, of course, is to select the correct model for the particular hospital that will enable positive outcomes and minimize negative ones. As stated before, whichever road is taken will commit a hospital for probably the next two to three years at least. The market is evolving, society is changing, our expectations of managed care are different than they were just last year. By the end of the decade, the hospital may discover, suddenly or slowly, that it has made an error. But by then, it may be too late to switch directions. And in which direction does it then go? That will not necessarily be clear, either. To avoid this dilemma as much as possible, it is absolutely critical that the healthcare executive team understand in intimate detail the following parameters:

The market

- the level of managed care penetration (what time frame will force action?);
- the status of key services and who provides them;
- where the market is going;
- what opportunities exist; and
- what minefields are waiting to be detonated.

The hospital

- the understanding of the new medical care paradigm by the board and top management, including medical management;
- an honest appraisal of the quality and kinds of services rendered (which can be tough if a pet program or high-profile clinical department is at stake);
- relationships with other area hospitals; and
- the capital available for any new venture.

The medical staff

- their commitment to the institutions, including their competing loyalties to others;
- potential leaders and champions among the staff (are they future physician executives within a new network structure?);
- the level of contribution of the individual practitioners and groups to the hospital and apparent trends regarding their practice patterns; and
- a reasonable prediction of what to expect from the staff when change finally arrives (this concerns first and foremost autonomy issues).

The external environment

- who are the players in the market;
- what are their strategic objectives and how do those objectives affect the network under development;
- what is the regulatory scene in the state; and
- what effect will the movement of large numbers of Medicare and Medicaid members into managed care have on the market and the organization?

Several thick binders can be filled easily by a study team devoted to answering these points. There are many not listed that are also relevant to a particular case. The risk is that such a binder will find its place on the shelf in the conference room, never to be opened again after the formal presentation to management. This is an all-too-common occurrence. Yet it is indispensable preparation. "Measure twice, cut once." In healthcare strategic planning, this old saying should probably be "measure ten times, then act—but don't wait too long."

Lessons for the Healthcare Executive

Beyond the initial analysis, represented by the action list above, the executive team needs to perform a careful strategic evaluation of options. I will leave it to the reader to dust off the books from business school that discuss threats, opportunities, weaknesses, strengths, BGE analysis, Porter's matrix, etc. These are truly useful tools that have proven their worth in a variety of settings. Yet I am amazed constantly at how frequently healthcare organizations are willing to sink millions of dollars into projects that have not undergone any sort of rigorous analysis. It is a reminder of how the healthcare industry has been sheltered from the real-world economic forces that have taught other industries to utilize these concepts to evaluate a business decision *before* the check is written. In medicine, we have had the luxury of sloth and have been slow, if not resistant, to addressing our inefficiencies. For the organization that is cognizant of this deficit, there is a golden chance to gain the high ground in the market by being that much more prepared and informed than one's competitors. It is also an excellent way to demonstrate value to employers who look on the strategic planning process as a prerequisite to any type of venture. They have yet to fathom why healthcare providers do not do this routinely.

First, we must embrace the concept of the hospital as purely a *cost center*. It has been a revenue center for most of the last century, since the rise of the modern hospital. But as part of a network devoted to rational allocation of services and resources, this mind-set can cause havoc. An excellent example is the delivery of chemotherapy. Cancer patients are receiving ever-larger portions of their chemo regimens in physicians' offices (National Cancer Institute 1996). This has meant the loss of this revenue to hospital inpatient and outpatient departments. In the larger context of the network, however, this becomes a locus of competitive focal segmentation. The network can offer the payor ambulatory chemo services, with the benefits of lower costs. (I assume the oncologists follow the network's goal of providing care at a lower cost than the hospital usually does and so do not charge excessive fees; this has been a problem in some localities when office-based chemotherapy is mistakenly exempted from cost analysis by the network.)

There is also an important customer satisfaction component, with more convenience for the patient who can often combine chemo treatments with office visits. The patient is able to maintain self-sufficiency and be productive at work for a longer period of time. This is the kind of outcome that really matters to employers. The revenue loss to the hospital rolls into a net gain for the network. It also will probably lead to an indirect gain for the hospital as the oncologist generates more business because the network can secure and service contracts, sending some of that increased income to hospital-sponsored services (lab, outpatient testing, etc.). By focusing on the larger picture, both the network and the hospital realize a benefit.

This is directly related to the second point. One must ask: Who does the administrative structure of the network reflect? In hospital-sponsored networks, the hospital has the cash, the information systems (primitive as they may be), the infrastructure, and at least some knowledge of business principles. As a result, an HSN tends to look an awful lot like the hospital(s) forming it. There is frequently no physician executive at a senior decision-making level (a chronic complaint I have raised in this discussion, but for a reason). The character of the network takes on major significance as the HSN moves from planning to implementation. It is then that the HSN needs to demonstrate to potential customers that it can indeed achieve the savings, quality indicators (such as Health Employer Data and Information Set [HEDIS] criteria), and medical management goals. Both with the merger (centralized control) and alliance (decentralized) frameworks, this is a tall order. Further, one must always be aware that perception is reality: If the physicians and payors perceive the HSN to be a creature of the hospitals, with physicians as an add-on after the fact, the credibility of the network will suffer.

This obviously means intense communication with medical staffs. It also means talking to the health plans and finding out what they want. It is astonishing how rarely this is done by providers, as if the bureaucratic facade of an HMO or MCO is impenetrable by human contact. The HSN may have a rather different view of what the market is demanding. The leadership of the network may be pleasantly surprised at how willing the MCO may be to tell them *exactly* what to do to win their business (van Amerongen 1997). A good example of employers sharing their needs with providers, and thereby sparking a new initiative, is the development of managed worker's compensation programs ("managed comp"). For decades, hospitals measured their success in treating trauma using the standard indicators of length of stay, morbidity, and mortality. But what is important to employers (especially as global case rates reduce the variations in charges for classes of medical and surgical treatments) is when the employee will return to work and at what level of productivity. If the person will not be able to return, what will be the level of functionality and what resources will be required to support that person in the home? Within the past two years, a plethora of companies (many sponsored by MCOs, others by rehab centers and providers) has blossomed to meet this need. The farsighted HSN accurately identifies such opportunities and moves proactively to seize them.

Third, every network should critically assess how it will benefit the community. The primary purpose of any business initiative is to benefit the company and its customers. But in healthcare we must be constantly aware of the larger community. One of the flaws of our fee-for-service system has been the ability of substandard providers to continue to function, soaking up resources and delivering marginal or even poor care. The rush to consolidate and form networks, sometimes driven by panic, often leads to a failure to consider the ultimate effects on the community (as distinct from the market). This is another way of asking if this project really makes sense. Is the need there for a network, beyond the self-interest of the hospital to do something to stir up business? If this litmus test had been more frequently applied in the past, we might not now find so many areas overflowing with unused hospital beds (*Baltimore Sun* 1995). Conversely, the network that *is* able to show this sort of added value for the community will not only be performing a positive good, but will have another source of differentiation from its competitors. It would also serve as a further enticement to physicians to cast their lots with the network and give it their strong support.

Last, practical matters must be attended to with the same vigor as developing a vision, establishing communication, educating physicians and customers, etc. Two such practical matters are contracting and choosing a CEO. Contracts must be on hand when going to payors for business or to physicians to secure their participation. This seems simple, but it is often neglected. The content and "user-friendly" nature of these documents must be addressed. More than one physician group has walked away from a potential relationship because the contracts seemed one-sided or unfair. Prices must be reasonable and accurately reflect the services performed and resources consumed (*Modern Healthcare* 1997e). These prices must be in line with the other healthcare providers. All of this requires research and a willingness to negotiate. The fears of the practitioners must be allayed.

The issue of physician executives has been presented in several different ways. But what of the CEO of the network itself, assuming he or she is not a doctor? The trap here is to search so diligently for the "perfect" candidate that the network does not receive the guidance it must have in the formative stages. In the experience of a rural western network that eventually failed, the absence of a champion ultimately prevented the HSN from gaining physician support. It was unable to compete effectively with a local independent practice association that was able to locate and put in place a vibrant leader, not necessarily one with extensive experience (*Modern Healthcare* 1997d). The lesson to be learned is that it is better to have an energetic, enthusiastic CEO who can overcome inexperience than to lose valuable momentum by allowing the corporation to drift without a leader.

Lessons for Physicians

It should be clear by now that most hospitals have concluded that networks of physicians and hospitals will be a cornerstone of the medical delivery system going forward. These networks must add value to the tasks now done by hospitals alone. They must create an infrastructure that will allow the new combination of "hospital + physician" to present itself as operationally viable to payors. Physicians are therefore at the confluence of the network movement and have an enlarging role to play. The medical community has unfortunately been reticent to step forward and accept this responsibility. Their resistance to change, exemplified by the bitter opposition to Medicare in the early 1960s, is legendary. (In one amazing gesture, the AMA rented Madison Square Garden and packed it with doctors and their office staffs who listened as AMA officials delivered blistering attacks on the new government program. The irony, of course, is that Medicare has become the financial salvation of many physicians—and hospitals [*Modern Physician* 1997].)

This trend is, happily, changing. As more doctors take an interest in the business aspects of medical practice, aside from their traditional roles as small businessmen (*Modern Physician* 1997), medicine is looking less like a cottage industry. The challenge for physician executives is to become more actively and vocally involved in network formation. This must occur at the very start of the process, not downstream after critical decisions have already been made. It means moving beyond the fee-for-service mind-set and accepting the reality of the new medical landscape. This can be as much of a cultural change, with its attendant upheavals, as those discussed in the context of merging hospitals and combining their differing cultures. Once done, this cultural change will give the physicians who can do it a huge advantage over their peers in being able to affect their future. Without this understanding, irrelevance will quickly overtake the medical groups that try to continue to practice in the old patterns of the fee-for-service world.

A second lesson for physician executives is to move past the physician-hospital organization (PHO). The product life cycle (PLC) demonstrates why this is a priority for physicians who want to stay ahead of the wave and not behind it. The PLC is a measure of how a product (or a service) survives over time (Duncan 1995). It is based on the principle that all products, and even ideas, go through several distinct phases, or stages. These stages tend to relate to the shifting nature of the market as well as tastes, trends, technological advances, etc. Four stages are identified: introductory, growth, maturity, and decline. Figure 2.1 represents the PLC for hospitals. The unique characteristic is the length of the growth and maturity phases, each lasting several decades. It has outlasted many other industries and has been in a period of stability for a generation. Only recently, with the inclination toward outpatient and ambulatory care and the growing influence of MCOs, have hospitals begun to see a decline (although profits for hospitals continue to be robust [Virginia Department of Health 1996]).

The diagram I would propose for PHOs is very different. Stage II, growth, was phenomenally rapid as PHOs exploded onto the scene. Every hospital had to have one, and every doctor felt an almost irresistible

Figure 2.1 Product Life Cycle

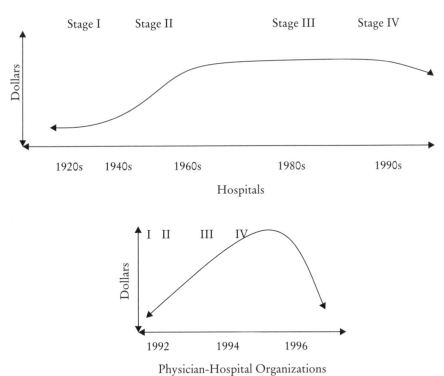

pressure to sign up with them all. But almost as soon as this wave crested, it began to fall as HSNs and other networks appeared. Payors became wary of PHOs almost from the start, with concerns about their ability to implement managed care principles within the setting of an open access (for physicians) plan. Little discipline was in evidence, and observers were not convinced that a PHO was in a position to make tough decisions on medical management or difficult choices on network composition.

The upshot is a retreat from the PHO model on the part of the hospitals, a retreat that should be noticed by physicians. It should also be emulated by them. The more rigorous HSN model is rapidly replacing the PHO one. Although moribund, many PHOs persist and physicians should avoid devoting any of their precious time or attention to them. Their efforts should be directed to gaining that seat at the HSN table (or whatever network option they decide to pursue, as will be discussed later). For, in addition to being eclipsed on a business level by the more intense network formation activity, PHOs are limiting their potential for success by failing to support the necessary redistribution of policy and income away from the hospital and specialty care providers and toward primary care (Kongstvedt 1996). Primary care is what MCOs and employers want. (Recall the admonition in the advice to healthcare executives to talk to the customer. It is good advice for doctors as well who have often purposely isolated themselves from this source of information.) The principles of primary care—prevention, health promotion, a holistic approach to illness—are also those of managed care and of caring for a population (versus caring for an individual). Whatever impedes this redistribution cannot survive in the new medical environment.

The primary care-specialty care (PCP-SCP) conflict has been stoked by the changes in Medicare reimbursement that increase payments to PCPs at the direct expense of SCPs (*Wall Street Journal* 1997d). This is, of course, a major challenge to HSNs as well. They must be exceedingly careful not to fall into the trap of being a shill for the specialist-dominated medical staff. It bears repeating that insurers and employers are turning into very sophisticated purchasers. Their medical directors are well aware of the historical dynamics of hospital medical staffs, especially since many of them spent years on those very staffs. HSNs that cannot resolve the PCP-SCP conflict in favor of a product with a primary care flavor, capable of achieving specialty utilization targets, will wither on the vine. The latest trend in employer requests of health plans in fact is to have practice profiles of individual specialists sent to all of the PCPs in the network in order to more directly influence referral behavior by having the PCPs steer clear of high-cost SCPs.

This is exactly the kind of detailed cost- and quality-based decision making payors will be looking for to separate the serious candidates from the rest when shopping for a network. The skilled physician executive will be invaluable in sorting out this problem for the HSN, as well as communicating these new requirements to the PCPs and SCPs. Referral patterns remain a fatal defect for the PHO, set up as most were in a hasty reaction to events not well understood at the time.

Future Trends for HSNs

Assuming they survive (and this may require at least a small leap of faith), HSNs will transition from their current form to another. This is analogous to the evolutionary path being trod by managed care as well. Much of this is being driven by the shifting characteristics of what consumers are demanding. Now that the rising trend in healthcare costs has temporarily leveled off (*Wall Street Journal* 1997d), there is a growing chorus asking for both open access to providers (i.e., wide choice with few restrictions) and economic discipline (Goldsmith and Goran 1996). The pressure toward broad, all-inclusive networks is intense and has seriously affected such systems as Kaiser and Group Health (Goldsmith and Goran 1996). The movement seems to be in the direction of even future consolidation to meet this desire on the part of both purchasers and patients. The "integrated delivery system" has become a code phrase for this end point. However, I think there are significant reasons to move cautiously in this direction.

Beware the IDS!

The integrated delivery system (IDS) is a page torn from the history of industrial organizations. Since it made sense at one time for IBM and GM, why not for healthcare? The vision of a seamless delivery system, with patients, physicians, and information flowing freely between the components, is an attractive one. It is a vision that has sparked huge spending sprees by hospitals as they attempt to integrate vertically and horizontally. But just as IBM ran up against the shoals of readjustment in business theory, the IDS is not the panacea it may appear.

Consider a prime focus of IDS activity: the purchasing of physician practices. This is frequently seen as a shortcut to HSN formation. What could be simpler? Buy the doctors and specialists in the geographic areas needed to assemble a network, glue them to the hospital and its clinics and *voilà*: an IDS! The reality is a bit different. From the University of Pennsylvania to Columbia/HCA, many of these acquisitions have turned out badly (*Wall Street Journal* 1997f). The reasons are unexpectedly high expenses and declines in physician productivity. According to a Coopers & Lybrand survey reported in the *Wall Street Journal*, on average hospitals were incurring $97,000 in annual losses per acquired physician (1997f). Bringing on large numbers of doctors makes the reporting of outcomes, utilization figures, etc., critical, but it is something most hospital systems are not equipped to do. If the practice is outside the usual service area for the hospital/HSN, it is less likely physicians will redirect their patients to the new owner. Furthermore, buying a practice does not mean patients' health plans will allow them to use that facility. Putting physicians on salary or an income guarantee usually leads to a drop in productivity of 4 to 15 percent (*Wall Street Journal* 1997f).

Aside from salary, there are few monetary incentives that physicians can be offered to increase patient flow to the IDS. Columbia/HCA is under close scrutiny by federal investigators over its economic links to providers, including its physician investors (*Wall Street Journal* 1997e).

An important motivator for forming an IDS is to lower costs. But this is not necessarily what happens in reality. Consider the example of Humana, which tried to vertically integrate salaried physicians with its hospitals and insurance company (Herzlinger 1997). Humana was faced with running three different businesses simultaneously, two of which were new. Lower than expected referrals to the hospitals occurred at the same time physician productivity fell. The hospitals, the original focal point of the Humana system, experienced increased costs and reduced morale; they were no longer the "stars." The only way for Humana to survive as an HMO was to sell off its hospitals (giving a jump-start to a little company known as Columbia). In this case, an IDS did nothing to accomplish either the clinical or financial objectives of integration and was actually counterproductive.

Other examples are easy to find. Minneapolis is a pioneering center of managed care. If the IDS concept is to work anywhere, it should work well there. Yet Allina Health Systems has found it a struggle to act as an integrated company and balance a health plan, hospitals, and providers (*Modern Healthcare* 1997b). Ironically, in a city with a high managed care penetration, it is the hospitals that performed well and the diversified business component that dragged down profits. Allina also had difficulty finding appropriate incentives for physicians (*Modern Healthcare* 1997b).

There are multiple financial, organizational, and legal issues with IDS formation that should give pause before one moves beyond networks to be all things to all people. In the legal arena, antitrust concerns will become more important as consolidation pushes toward the IDS (*Modern Healthcare* 1997c). Creation of a dominant health system, not simply a comprehensive network with good geographical coverage, is likely to draw the attention of state regulators. This is especially true in smaller markets where the merger of several hospitals, the acquisition of some large group practices, and the marriage of competing health plans offered by those systems results in the possible violation of antitrust statutes.

Does the IDS create a culture that is supportive of innovation? This will be a vital characteristic of future successful systems. The dynamism of managed care change will demand new and increasingly creative solutions. Just two years ago, a request by an employer for a health plan to offer expanded choice while holding down costs would have seemed completely contradictory. Today, plans are scrambling to devise an answer. So much energy is consumed within an IDS in supporting the functions of that huge structure that little may be left for innovation. On the hospital side, the marginal cost of an inpatient day has fallen so far that owning hospitals within a health plan no longer makes sense (Goldsmith and Goran 1996). The large sums needed to acquire hospitals then burden the IDS with debt. In many respects, this is a classic case of "make or buy." The IDS is the medical equivalent of Henry Ford's original idea to have every piece of the Model T made by Ford Motor Company. In

Anti-Trust Acts Relevant to Healthcare: A Brief Discussion

The concept of market power is critical to Section 1 and Section 2 claims of the Sherman Anti-Trust Act. The plaintiff (for example, the state attorney general) must prove the defendant has "market power" under Section 1 claims. Section 2 prohibits monopolization and attempts to monopolize. The definition of a *market* for discerning market power requires two determinations: What is the relevant product market? What is the relevant geographic market?

Section 7 of the Clayton Act prohibits mergers and acquisitions where the effects may be to lessen competition substantially or create a monopoly. This act significantly affects merger cases.

Section 5 of the Federal Trade Commission Act prohibits unfair methods of competition and unfair deceptive acts or practices.

Bottom line: The law is meant to foster competition and fair trade practices in order to benefit the public. There is no presumption that the competition engendered will benefit the competitors. Unless a hospital or physician can show that the public is harmed by the new HMO or network in town, it is unlikely to be considered a violation of the antitrust laws, even if the new player threatens to do harm to competitors in the market; that is seen as beneficial to the consumer and a consequence of the competitive free market (Furrow 1991).

the 1990s, the auto industry is predicated upon outsourcing, searching out best-of-breed, and buying the competencies they need. Much is done outside the company and brought in or bought as needed. This concept is also a shift away from the philosophy of self-sufficiency that has had a long history in medicine. Only recently have hospitals accepted the notion that they can exist without having a department representing every possible branch of medicine.

A lesson begins to emerge from these bits of experience. The IDS is an answer to a question that was asked many years ago. The problem is that it has been replaced by a new question whose subtle differences are terribly important. We have progressed from "How can *we* deliver seamless care?" to "How can the *patient* receive seamless care?" Reframing the question in this manner points us in a different direction. Rather than fixating on binding up all the elements of healthcare into one package, the impetus is to find the proper dynamic between these elements. It may well be that the ideal mix is to "virtually" integrate components to achieve maximum functionality. This concept of virtual integration was promoted by Jeff Goldsmith (1996). Developing a web of agreements, protocols, and incentives, a framework is built that can effectively improve care and conserve clinical resources. It implies a method of having the pieces working together so they would appear seamless to the client (patient or payor). Yet the ownership and maintenance does not necessarily rest in one locus. This "learning system" framework would promote the innovation essential to the constant improvement required by the external environment. This ongoing process can work best only if the people with specialized knowledge—core competencies—are encouraged to frequently "step outside the box." When the box becomes large and ponderous (a sort of medical Pentagon), this simply will not happen. We see the small, nimble Silicon Valley companies constantly reinventing themselves and their products to respond to new trends. Despite the relentless change that whipsaws the high-tech industry, the successful companies still are able to integrate in a virtual fashion that is invisible to the customer, yet is remarkably effective. The challenge in healthcare is to invent similarly effective interfaces between our various components, but to do so without taking on the burdens inherent in the IDS.

In short, I see the IDS as a colossus waiting to tumble to earth. The trauma to the constituents when that occurs will be substantial and will retard their progress to the next stage of managed care. Likewise, HSNs, as they grow and acquire, run the same risk even if they do not achieve IDS status. It was stated earlier that we are really on the threshold of the future of managed care. We are misled if we view it as a done deed. We are definitely "not there yet." Physicians and healthcare executives have gone through some momentous transitions with the birth of these new ways of packaging and delivering services. It is unclear if HSNs will have a long-term future. But it is plain that PHOs are "dead men walking."

The final, fundamental problem with the IDS is that it does not address the future role of the hospital. Downsizing has only begun to occur. It will accelerate dramatically in the near term. As technology becomes available outside the hospital walls (witness the freestanding, investor-owned imaging centers), hospitals have lost their monopoly in this critical area. Fewer physicians want or need hospital privileges as more care becomes exclusively ambulatory. Whither, then, the hospital? It will occupy far less of a central position in our thinking about medical delivery issues. It continues to move from a revenue center to a cost center. But at the heart of the HSN is the hospital. Is the HSN prepared to see the hospital component diminish? The answer is probably no, and it will provoke a new flurry of reactionary activity as it comes to pass. The source of new delivery paradigms, the ones that will last into the next decades and set the stage for what is to follow, lies elsewhere. It is in the practitioner side of the equation that we shall see the real promise for understanding the twenty-first-century delivery system.

References

Backanavage, S. R., T. J. Lyons. 1997. "Hospitals and Managed Care." *American Journal of Managed Care* 3: 293–97.

Baltimore Sun. 1995. 11 November: 10.

Budget Report of the American Association of Medical Colleges. 1995. Washington, DC.

Callahan, J. J., D. S. Shepard, R. N. Beinecke, M. J. Larson, and D. Cavanaugh. 1995. "Mental Health and Substance Abuse Treatments in Managed Care: The Massachusetts Medicaid Experience." *Health Affairs* 14 (3): 173–84.

Christianson, J., B. Dowd, J. Kralewski, S. Hayes, and C. Wisner. 1995. "Managed Care in the Twin Cities: What Can We Learn?" *Health Affairs* 14 (2): 114–30.

Cincinnati Enquirer. 1997. "Hospital Beds Go Begging." 30 August: 1.

Clay, Peter. 1995a. Interview by author. 7 November.

———. 1995b. Interview by author. 12 December.

Duncan, J. 1995. *Strategic Management of Health Care Organizations.* Cambridge, MA: Blackwell Publishers.

Elwood, P. M. 1996. "How Doctors Can Regain Control of Health Care." *Medical Economics* June: 50–61.

Furrow, B. R. 1991. *Health Law.* St. Paul: West Publishing.

Goldsmith, J., and M. J. Goran. 1996. "Managed Care Mythology: Supply-Side Dreams Die Hard." *Health Care Forum Journal* November/December: 42–47.

Gray, B. H. 1991. *The Profit Motive and Patient Care.* Cambridge, MA: Harvard University Press.

Greene, J. 1997. "Does Integration Really Cut Costs?" *Modern Healthcare* 10 February: 34–40.

Herzlinger, R. 1997. "Retooling Health Care." *Modern Healthcare* 14 February: 96.

Inglehart, J. K. 1997. "Listening in on the Duke University Private Sector Conference." *New England Journal of Medicine* 336: 1827–31.

Kassirer, J. P. 1996. "Mergers and Acquisitions: Who Benefits? Who Loses?" *New England Journal of Medicine* 334: 722–23.

Kongstvedt, P. 1996. *The Managed Care Handbook.* Gaithersburg, MD: Aspen Publishers.

Life. 1969. 7 March: 12.

Managed Healthcare. 1997. "Oxford's Dream Team." December: 36–38.

Medical Herald. 1995. "Doctor/Hospital Network Upsets Insurers." 5 (10): 23.

Modern Healthcare. 1995a. "Alliances Have New Strategy." 10 July: 34.

———. 1995b. "Networks: The Chicago Archdiocese Experience." 1 November: 7.

———. 1995c. "Too Many Beds in Baltimore." 10 July: 6.

———. 1997a. 7 February: 14.

———. 1997b. "PA Link in Works." 17 February: 30–32.

———. 1997c. "Anti-Trust Concerns Slow PA Merger." 30 June: 2.

———. 1997d. "Failed Rural Washington Network Lacked Physician Support." 30 June: 140.

———. 1997e. "Indiana Hospital Sticks to Guns on Fair Pricing." 30 June: 106.

————. 1997f. "The Doc's the Anchor." 30 June: 38.

Modern Physician. 1997. "This Time, Seize the Opportunity." May: 12.

National Cancer Institute. 1996. *Cancer Facts.* Bethesda, MD.

New York Times. 1997. "A Low Price for Better Health Care." 29 June: C1.

Phelps, C. E. 1992. *Health Economics.* New York: HarperCollins.

Roggy, S., and R. Gorrity. 1993. "Bridging the Visions of Competing Catholic Health Care Systems." *Health Care Strategic Management* 11: 16–19.

"The GE Health Care Preferred Scorecard Manual." 1997. Fairfield, CT.

University of Minnesota Health Research Center. *Rural Health Networks.* 1996.

van Amerongen, D. 1996. "Survey of CEOs and Medical Staff Presidents in the Atlantic Health Alliance." Management application paper, University of Wisconsin Department of Administrative Medicine.

————. 1997. "The Rush to Consolidate and the Future of Medical Practice." *Physician Executive* 23 (1): 4–8.

Virginia Department of Health. 1996. *Buyers Guide to Efficient and Productive Hospitals and Nursing Homes.*

Wachter, R. M., and L. Goldman. 1996. "The Emerging Role of 'Hospitalists' in the American Health Care System." *New England Journal of Medicine* 335: 514–17.

Wall Street Journal. 1995. "Chrysler Is Ending Long Relationship under which Mitsubishi Supplied Cars." 16 October: 10.

————. 1997a. 25 January: A3.

————. 1997b. 18 February: B2.

————. 1997c. 16 June: A1.

————. 1997d. "Health-Cost Trims Hold Inflation Down." 30 June: A1.

————. 1997e. "Hospital-Doctor Ties Can Be a Legal Quagmire." 27 April: B1.

————. 1997f. "Hospitals That Gobbled up Physician Practices Fell Ill." 19 June: B6.

3

PROVIDER-SPONSORED NETWORKS

"Shall I say in the future:
1. You are too bad a risk; go to a first-class surgeon;
2. You are too bad a risk; I must double my usual fee;
3. You are too bad a risk; you need not pay me unless you live.
All are logical. I like the last best."
—Ernest Codman, M.D., pioneer of quality assurance in surgery, 1915

THIS IS the most traumatic period in this century for the practicing physician. The message often perceived by the doctor in the office in the community, trying as best as possible to care for patients, is that "Everything you know is wrong." The shifts we are all experiencing are huge. I would argue they are more profound than at other times because the changes reach deeper. There have been other occasions when significant adjustments in medical practice took place: the use of the hospital-aligned physician, the expansion of specialties after World War II, the advent of third-party payors. But only managed care has so fundamentally affected the way every American perceives, receives, and pays for healthcare. As Uwe Reinhardt of Princeton says, "The keys to the treasury are being taken away" (Carlson 1997).

But this goes beyond just financial issues. Previous changes have never been a composite of financial, ethical, philosophical, and medical realignments, with entirely new concepts such as quality improvement and accountability thrown in as well. For physician executives and health-care executives who have recently joined the work force, this is less of an issue. They have been "raised" on the turmoil of the last 10 to 15 years; it is part of their formation as healthcare workers. For those much older, it is also less of a problem, since retirement in the next several years will resolve this for them. The mid-career physician, physician executive, and healthcare executive—who entered medicine in the heyday of fee-for-service laissez-faire and still have many years of contributions to make—find their new scenario far more daunting.

"Anxiety caused by change can only be cured by more change," says a proverb. The approach, however, of organized medicine to most elements of managed care has been to fight a rear-guard action, sniping at the edges, promoting a "return" to the old fee-for-service system. It has converted the American Medical Association, the *New England Journal of Medicine*, and others into the "nattering nabobs of negativism" Spiro Agnew loved to condemn. Their unrestrained criticism of managed care is usually done in a vacuum, with no recognition of the antecedents of our current healthcare crisis or any sort of positive solution other than to resume the status quo (*Medical Economics* 1997). Even when the representatives of managed care have attempted to address their criticism and incorporate it into new initiatives, it is often bitterly attacked as not being good enough, fast enough, etc. (Kassirer 1997). The purpose of the critics thus becomes more to stall reform than to help shape it.

This comes at a potential cost. By refusing to meet managed care halfway, these opponents run the risk of marginalizing themselves in the debate. Employees expect to enroll nearly 40 percent of their workers in HMOs by 2000, up 31 percent from 1997, despite the backlash against managed care (*Wall Street Journal* 1997b). The 1997 Budget Accord in Congress included specific strategies for increasing enrollment in Medicare HMOs (*Cincinnati Enquirer* 1997). The momentum is clearly there for those who choose to see it. This would seem to be an era of declining dominance for physicians as the drivers of the medical care system, yet the trends I see tell a radically different tale. Rather than watching the eclipse of physician power, we are on the threshold of a golden, almost historic, opportunity for physicians to regain predominance in medicine they have not known in this century. Such an outcome is available to those farsighted physicians and groups who have the tools and skills necessary to take advantage of this opportunity.

How to accomplish this is the subject of this chapter. It is important to keep in mind the themes of this book discussed at length in Chapter 1. Among them were understand your competencies and focus on them, gain power by accepting reality, and acknowledge the direction this country's medical care is taking and figure out how to be a part of it. The result will be a winning solution that will accomplish several ends: it will be financially rewarding; it will be professionally satisfying; and it will actually, at the end of the day, help people to receive the care they deserve. For physicians and healthcare executives outside the hospital setting, the vehicle to achieve this is the provider-sponsored network (PSN).

What Is a PSN?

The definition of a PSN is important to understand clearly. A great deal of confusion exists between HSNs and PSNs. Many hospitals would be quite happy for their affiliated HSNs to be tagged by the world at large as being provider-sponsored. But to be a PSN, with an independent strategy, requires true sponsorship by physicians, with physician leadership. Figure 3.1 illustrates these differences. Only when the resources for the PSN are really derived from the physicians' side can a network even be considered a PSN.

A set of criteria to identify a PSN more easily, and to be used as a road map for implementation, is given in Table 3.1. The issue of physician leadership is just and foremost. The motivation must emanate with physicians, such that the purpose of the PSN is centered on the mission of being a vehicle to accomplish the objectives that create a

Figure 3.1   Etiologic Differences Between HSNs and PSNs

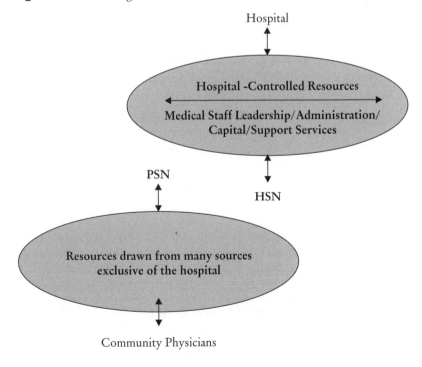

Table 3.1 Criteria Defining a Physician-Sponsored Network

1. Visionary physician leadership
2. An existence outside the context of the hospital
3. A common set of behaviors, extending beyond financial issues and involving a new pattern of care
4. Unity of purpose
5. An ambulatory perspective
6. Service experience

physician-centered delivery system. This may sound like a PHO, or an HSN that has given a prominent role to a physician executive, but it is qualitatively different. Only by starting on the physician side (read ambulatory, multi-site, community-based) does the PSN acquire the true nature of being organized around, and for, doctors. This leadership must be visionary. It is not enough for physicians to band together simply to achieve economies of scale. There are other, less involved ways to take advantage of buying in bulk. Rather, the leadership must have a vision of how the PSN can add value to the community. This involves identifying needs, understanding trends, and then meeting them. These dimensions are summarized in Table 3.2.

This leads to the second criterion: the PSN exists completely *outside* the context of the hospital. This does not simply refer to physical location. A PHO or HSN may well have its offices remote from the hospital campus, yet still be joined at the hip. A true PSN must make that switch from seeing the hospital as a resource center and instead view it as a cost-generator. The hospital, even one that may be dominant in the community with a long history of being the "hub in the wheel" of the local medical delivery system, becomes one of several possible vendors of services to the PSN. This is admittedly not an easy mental shift to

Table 3.2 Dimensions of the Visionary Physician Leader

1. Communicates the vision of the network within the context of the new healthcare paradigm and promotes confidence in the medical mission of the network
2. Understands organizational behavior, including how organizations grow and mature
3. Manages physicians: aligning incentives, addressing issues of autonomy, and helping the medical group move beyond the traditional view of the medical system
4. Fosters a philosophy of continuous quality improvement from the top down and expresses this commitment to quality to customers and patients
5. Focuses on solving problems with available resources and getting the job done; has a positive attitude toward change and the challenges to be met

make. For the past 70 years, physicians have functioned as satellites to the hospital. For the past 35 years of Medicare and Medicaid, the hospital piece was a major part of the revenue stream of the average practitioner. It is traumatic to picture the end of this symbolic relationship, but I believe farsighted medical groups will understand this trend and position themselves accordingly.

The PSN is defined by a common set of behaviors. Ideally this is what has always brought physicians together—the desire to practice a particular type or philosophy of medicine with others of the same mind. As most familiar with medical practice know, the ideal is seldom realized. The group practice model became more of a business model than a medical one. Five names might be on the door, but five different approaches to care performed under that one roof. (I well remember patients who would receive radically different care depending on which doctor went off or came on call each morning.) Very little room exists for such variation in the managed care setting. Much of what has led companies to embrace managed care is the drive to eliminate the kind of differences in treatment that they are able to chart.

"Modifying physician behavior" has become the rallying cry of all, including the government. While a segment of the medical establishment sees this as a threat, it is in fact a golden door waiting to be opened. Under the strong leadership of a visionary physician executive, a common mission and objectives are written. Hopefully, the team (and it must be a *team* led by the physician leader[s]) starts with a blank sheet of paper and attacks the challenge to design a new pattern of care. This approach is a big departure from simply reworking the status quo. Yet it can lead, with surprisingly straightforward logic, to a common set of operating standards. These standards in turn can provide the impetus for group members to question previous behavior, understand how altering it can result in better care and a more effective practice, and help them to meet the expectations of their new customers: patients/members, health plans, and employers. This change is powerful. It can communicate to both the internal world of practice (the physicians and staff) and the external world of potential customers that the group is ready to do business. Only when these values are shared by the entire group will behavior really be modified. This transforms the group from just a bunch of doctors, trying to save money by sharing a nurse, into a true coordinated medical practice (Marr 1997).

It is essential that the vision and mission of the PSN extend beyond simply making money or "keeping up with Dr. Jones." A true sense of purpose must motivate the group. Those external to the practice need to understand the motivation of the group, just as the group members do. Once their ethos is part of the makeup of the PSN, learning the needed behaviors becomes much more feasible. The lesson for physician and healthcare executives is that financial goals alone do not address unity of purpose. This too is part of the definition of a PSN. Cohesion among the members is critical. It is appropriate that physicians who are trying to build something that is larger than the group itself will come together more effectively. Efficiency is a hallmark of a good group practice; effectiveness is the hallmark of a PSN that is attractive to employees and payors.

The PSN functions from an ambulatory perspective. This orientation reconfigures the entire nature of the medical care delivered. As mentioned, it reduces the hospital (or inpatient piece) to the status of a vendor, rather than the chief component of care. The noninpatient services of a hospital system become less linked to the use of that hospital. The PSN, with its freedom of action independent of a given facility, can move easily to pick and choose which services to buy. This obviously appeals to payors who understand the value of choosing between competing suppliers in order to find the best price and service.

For an MCO, an additional attractive feature emerges. Care in the traditional system has always been fragmented. With a delivery system structured around a hospital, this fragmentation will never be entirely eliminated. While the PSN is not meant to be a magic bullet, its position is outside the bricks and mortar, hence closer to the patient. The perspective gained allows a longitudinal approach to patient care. This permits a PSN to incorporate preventive services, health maintenance services, acute and chronic care, and so on into its delivery model. Proponents of HSNs and PHOs will argue that their structures permit the same. But the mind-set of any system anchored, however indirectly, to a hospital cannot escape the point of view that places the patient as only a few steps away from a bed. This is a great advantage of the PSN in not being tied to using or supporting a particular facility. (Although this seems to be antihospital, I believe this trend will only accelerate. Furthermore, it will actually be beneficial for hospitals. As they are forced to compete, often against for-profit rivals, they will have to develop the efficiencies and know-how to provide more effective care, in more attractive ways, to purchasers. The lack of competition has been a major handicap for the hospital industry, one that is only recently being remedied. Developing new methods to satisfy PSN customers will only make them stronger.)

PSNs also have the potential to employ the experience of their physicians to provide value for their members and customers. It must be remembered that our chief product in medicine has always been service. It is continually fascinating to me as I work with large employers and medical organizations to see, as we near 2000, how we are coming full circle to a medical delivery model that existed in 1900. What are the concerns of employers about the healthcare they want for their thousands of employees? It is not how many computerized axial tomography (CT) scans are available or how many transplant centers exist; rather, it is how far is it to the nearest family doctor? How long do people have to wait in the office? Is it easy to get an appointment? How many women get Pap smears? These are low-tech, high-touch services, easily provided by a competent generalist. Yet they are valued very highly by purchasers—more so, ironically, than the technology.

The PSN that grasps this fact will be light-years ahead of its hospital-based counterpart. That is not to say that technology is not important. It has, however, come to be seen as a given. We expect cars to run well and be relatively maintenance free. Most marketing surveys show that technological components are the "price of admission" for a car to be considered by a customer. What sells it are the "feel," the "look," the service provided by the dealer (of course, most people still buy a car based on the cup holder). Likewise, the lay public (including multimillion dollar corporations) assumes a prospective provider offers high quality service, or else it would not be at the table in the first place. PSNs have a built-in advantage in their experience (through their physicians who make up the core of the network) to deliver their service piece that is so sought after by consumers. This is a somewhat vague concept, but I believe it is terribly important. In a marketplace that demands precise differentiation in order for consumers to choose properly, it can be a deciding factor.

Caveats for PSNs

PSNs create the opportunity for physicians to go back to the drawing board and redesign their patterns of care. This is an exciting crossroads for American medicine as we rediscover our roots in generalist, patient-focused, ambulatory care. Yet, there are caveats to this approach. Some are obvious from the preceding discussion. It is essential that a true PSN be the outcome of this process. Attempting to recast an HSN as a PSN, or to set up a facade for possible purchasers, is guaranteed to fail. Those who do not walk the walk and talk the talk will be quickly found out. Corporations and insurers are hiring full-time medical directors at an amazing clip. Corporate medical executives are well aware of what their companies are after and have sophisticated resources at their disposal to evaluate all suitors. The network leadership meeting for the first time with an interested corporate client must never delude itself into thinking that the medical knowledge is concentrated on its side of the negotiations. The era of asymmetry of information, at least in this context, is over.

The primary cause of many PSNs' downfall is in the desire to act as a payor. Frustration over managed care has led many a physician to wonder about circumventing the insurance companies and going straight to the employers. It is an appealing concept. By cutting out the "middle man," variance costs can be saved, a competitive price offered, and physicians can be reimbursed in a fee-for-service manner with less paperwork. We all tend to complain about the added costs and presumed inefficiencies imposed by intermediaries who do not seem to earn their portion of the pie. For physicians whose expertise is indispensable in providing care, this feeling is even more intense (Kuttner 1997). The problem with this argument is that it does not account for the complexity and demands of medical care delivery versus the practice of medicine one-on-one. The desire to be both payor and provider has rarely been successful. The infrastructure and resources required to perform the insurance function are usually beyond the ken of even the most astute physician executives. Up until the era of managed care, insurance revolved around premiums, paying claims, and an actuarial function that permitted the company to appropriately risk-adjust its product. In some respects this would have been the ideal time for physicians to take over the insurance end because of its relative simplicity compared to the present. Of course, 20 years ago physicians were still, as Reinhardt says, "holding the keys to the treasury" so there was no motivation to do so (Inglehart 1997).

Today, a managed care organization's obligation has eclipsed these straightforward ones. Information systems consume huge percentages of the company budget. It is necessary to provide detailed analysis of provider profiles, care trends, utilization of dozens of different services and procedures, drug usage, referrals, and so on. This data is needed not only for internal use but to report to regulatory bodies and to feed back to employers (who are demanding ever-more precise reporting on the costs and utilization of their covered groups). All of the various components of medical management also require major resources-demand management, care and case management, disease state management, and so on. Such activities are the tip of the iceberg for any payor, be it a Prudential, United Health Care, Sister of Charity, Blues Plan, or a PSN that wants to be a payor.

An illustrative example is appropriate at this point. Coastal Physicians Group was a pioneer in building networks of physician practices. It was widely profiled in the press and became a publicly traded company (Deogun 1996). As it grew, it spread into the HMO business. However, the company had few financial controls; acquisitions were not integrated; and subsidiaries used different financial systems. Data was not reported in a uniform manner. Financial reserves, required by state insurance regulations, were not always adequate. Pressure from other large HMOs, with deeper pockets and more experience, increased. Although the company is still in business, it has been racked by lawsuits, regulatory investigations, etc.

The question to ask at the end of the day is, Why do you want to set up this PSN? As I have tried to convey, the PSN whose focus is on reconfiguring medical care delivery with the physician as the heart of the system is the model that will stand the test of time. Aside from playing to the core competency of physicians, it has a clear and understandable vision for customers and patients. The other lesson is that any network designed as a reactive, financially driven response to market changes does not have a future. This is especially true for a PSN that does not have the capital resources of a hospital on which to draw.

PSNs and HSNs

When they are properly structured, PSNs have great potential. They have the tools to make themselves very attractive to purchasers. They possess inherent advantages over HSNs. Despite their drawbacks, HSNs may well continue to generate a low level of business for their sponsoring organizations. The trend I foresee, however, is for PSNs to surpass HSNs quickly as viable forces in the marketplace and to take over the "physician" chair at the negotiating table. It is important to have a full understanding of PSNs to discuss why this will happen.

HSNs, successors to PHOs, were to be the hospitals' method of supplying the physician piece of the puzzle. This has yet to materialize. Certainly, some HSNs have met with success. However, whatever accomplishments have been achieved are limited with respect to the energy and capital invested in the networks. Because of their basic nature, HSNs will not be able to compete with a fully functioning PSN. Table 3.3 highlights the differences between the two structures. First, few HSNs are selective. As we have seen, HSNs were almost a panicked response to increasing pressure. Payors wanted a network with a broad service area; hospitals simply rolled over their medical staffs into the new entity. A survey done of hospital-sponsored networks in central Maryland in 1995 showed only 1 of 17 hospitals in three networks did not incorporate its entire staff into the HSN (van Amerongen 1996). Selectivity will become a litmus test for networks going forward. The PSN is better positioned to perform this screening because it does not have an automatic obligation to every practitioner on the medical staff. The lack of selectivity means

Table 3.3   Compared to the PSN, the HSN:

- Is not selective in who is recruited to join the physician staff
- Is unable by the nature of its sponsoring entity to meaningfully reduce inpatient capacity and utilization
- Has an inherent conflict between the goals of the payor (to purchase cost-effective care in the most cost-efficient setting) and the goals of the sponsor (to increase hospital revenues and maximize use of the hospital facilities, the bulk of which are inpatient units)
- Has loose medical management
- Provides unencumbered capital to the participating physician groups

physicians will be recruited who are not compatible with the needs of a managed care network. Generally, these are low-quality physicians, physicians who are antagonistic to change, high-utilizing subspecialists, etc. Hopefully, the PSN will be able to identify such practitioners and guard against stacking their network with them. It must be remembered that preventing a physician from joining is a simple task compared to removing a participating provider from a network.

HSNs are designed, if only indirectly, to fill beds. The HSN's stated goal may be to function as an ambulatory group. Yet, the premise is that the patients of the network will access outpatient services provided by the hospital. This in turn means a certain percentage will end up admitted as inpatients. Profiles of physicians working for Columbia/HCA HSNs have shown drastic increases in admission to the Columbia hospitals (*New York Times* 1997). Even if the HSN does not "perform" to this level, nothing is done by the HSN to reduce excess capacity. For employers (as well as the government and insurers), the issue of too many beds and services is serious. Employers are aggressively moving into the community to understand at a precise level what drives utilization and costs. They know hospitals are not full, and they are interested in using their market power to reduce this excess. As a patient-centered, independent organization, the PSN has a built-in ability to look critically at various providers, choosing some and not others. The result will be increased pressure on the areas of redundant services, ultimately reducing them.

Once a contract is won, it must be serviced. In the managed care setting this translates into tight control of utilization. This causes a fundamental conflict between the contract and the sponsor of the network. How to resolve this conflict is unclear, and it may well be that it cannot be put to rest. Astute purchasers of healthcare know this and tend to put HSNs low on their list of prospects.

Managing physicians has been compared to herding cats. Doctors by nature and training are independent and self-reliant. Getting them to conform to a corporate standard is one of the greatest challenges of medical administration. Staff model HMOs have generally had difficulty bringing physicians into line. Even when they are employees, doctors tend to do what they will, leading some employer groups to rank staff-model HMOs last on the list of desirable partners (*Medical Interface* 1996). At the other extreme from the staff model is the HSN that acts at best as a contracting agent and virtually not at all as a shaper of physician behavior. Because of the loose management of the physicians, this type of HSN is unable to deliver any meaningful savings or reductions in variation to the customer. Assuming that HSNs would set up aggressive risk management with its members, one could postulate a positive swing in behavior. But this requires a strong physician leadership and the willingness to make some very tough political decisions—both of which tend to be absent in the HSN environment. Are they present in the PSN? Not necessarily. But the alternative of risk arrangements, presented by a strong physician champion, is far more likely. It will also be plain to any potential partner whether or not the PSN is serious about medical management.

Capital is often an overlooked issue as physicians decide which road to take. HSNs certainly tend to have a richer source of funds than PSNs. The example given earlier of the PSN in Pennsylvania that floundered because of a cash crunch is a telling one. Yet it is imperative to remember that an HSN's sources of capital may not be unencumbered. Several hospital systems have ended up burdening their HSNs with debt unintentionally because of the vagaries of capital transfers, the tax code, etc. (*Wall Street Journal* 1997a). For the individual practitioner, these behind-the-scenes machinations can be damaging. If the doctor has cast lots with the HSN, and even bought into it, such financial difficulties can stymie contracting and sink the physicians who are relying on the HSN to generate patient volume.

It is interesting to note that even without the capital resources available to most hospitals, the plurality of HMO contracts are not held by HSNs (see Figure 3.2). This graph should be disturbing news for hospital systems. Even with the infrastructure, capital, name recognition, and other supposed advantages that hospitals bring to their networks, they have been unable to capture the market. Logically one would expect the more organized player to dominate all other less-experienced competitors. That this has not happened speaks volumes for the future of HSNs.

While hospitals offer a source of capital, they also may be a source of debt. In Massachusetts, a hospital system wanted to position its HSN to win contracts. It was already saddled with $50 million in debt, and needed another $40–$50 million to make renovations to its facilities and place the HSN on a proper standing with sufficient reserves. The system turned to an outside partner that required a profit to be made before any money could be allotted: a classic catch-22. Hence, any physician group seeking to break into managed care via this HSN was frustrated by the hospital's internal financial difficulties that had nothing to do with the ability of those doctors to provide appropriate care to clients in their community (Peters 1988).

Hospital Strategies Beyond HSNs

Despite the failure of HSNs to catch on, hospitals continue to explore new means of linking with physicians. One recent example is the management service organization (MSO), the latest variation on the PHO/HSN theme. However, there are fundamental issues that prevent the vast majority of MSOs to succeed financially:

- problems balancing physician/hospital interests;
- inadequate information systems;
- "too many prior bad deals" (i.e., throwing good money after bad);

Figure 3.2 Estimates of HMO Contracts Held by Various Types of Delivery Systems in 1997

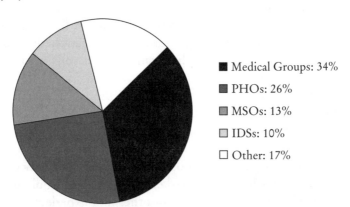

■ Medical Groups: 34%
■ PHOs: 26%
■ MSOs: 13%
□ IDSs: 10%
□ Other: 17%

Source: *OBG Management*, July 1997.

- no assistance for the physicians in learning about managed care;
- failure to track benchmark data;
- inability to share clinical data physician groups; and
- no electronic data exchange with the hospitals sponsors (Pallarito 1996).

This list could be a quick rendition of the problems with HSNs. It is also a warning to PSNs to pay attention to the traps that have kept HSNs from breaking into the new medical marketplace.

Integrated delivery systems (IDSs) represent another hospital-centered strategy. This approach seems to promote a vision of "seamless" care. In most contexts, it is presented as a coming together of physicians and facilities in one huge "silo" (another management buzzword) of care delivery. Recall the earlier comment that supporting IDSs mandates attention and resources. Further, it presumes that all care will be centered within the IDS silo. For patients with special needs, moving outside to another IDS disrupts the seamless aura. The Medimetrix review reminds us of the trouble hospitals have moving data from practice to hospital and back. This is unlikely to be any better between different (and competing) IDSs. The main point with regard to seamless care that is usually over-looked is that the care must appear seamless to the patient. Therefore, the optimal system will be designed to facilitate the patient moving from provider to provider easily, with the ability to identify and obtain the best services for a given situation.

The ideal scenario then becomes a patient-centered one, selecting among a variety of services that are matched to current needs, regard-less of where those services are located. (It reminds me of the tunnels underneath Walt Disney World that are invisible to the guests but allow Mickey to pop up at various places all over the park.) Considered in this light, we are brought once again to the PSN model, away from the PHO/HSN/MSO/IDS.

The take-home lesson is that the only point of view that really matters is that of the patient (and, secondarily, the employer or payor, but their opinion will be shaped by the patient's experience). The best system will be that which can mold itself to the patient's needs, rather than vice versa. This concept of seeing life from the patient's perspective is so frequently misunderstood in medical care that it may never have been considered when we started building these medical behemoths. How can we be customer-focused and flexible? Tom Peters, the management guru who helped kick-start the quality movement in the United States, speaks to this point in his book *Thriving on Chaos*. He describes a scenario in which dozens of different professionals came together over one weekend to produce a video for a large client. They established a working group, assigned tasks, dealt with problems as they arose, and remained focused on that job at hand. It was a unique job, requiring a unique combination of talent. After it was completed, the group disbanded. The various components of what had been, for a brief time, a highly specialized team concentrating on a complex problem, were then free to be configured for the demands of the next project (Covey 1990).

For physician and healthcare executives, this is a powerful lesson. It should be obvious by now that all successful strategies for the future will center on satisfying the customer. That customer may be an individual patient, an employer, HCFA, an insurer, or several of these components at once. Part of that satisfaction process is the ability to bend the system, align resources, or do whatever is necessary to meet the needs of a particular instance. The variety of situations is almost infinite. Hence the system that is willing and able to take on the challenge of creating a care pattern for a specific requirement will gain a tremendous advantage over competitors.

Physicians must realize that the era of expecting the patient and customer to change to meet *our* needs is over, as it well should be. The question then is what model permits such realignment of resources on a customized basis. This is the real power of the types of networks I have been suggesting. And though it is certainly possible to conceive of such a fluid process existing in the hospital context, it is far less likely that it can be realized. The very nature of the large, bureaucratic organization militates against it. Further, the more distance between the customer and the decision maker, the less responsive the occupation will be. This is another lesson Tom Peters teaches us. Why did Detroit take *so long* in the early 1980s to understand that Americans wanted smaller, more fuel-efficient cars like Hondas and Toyotas? It was mainly because most auto executives were white males who lived in the suburbs and drove large gas guzzlers. They could not conceive of people wanting something else. Likewise, I believe the experience of hands-on patient care that is part of the training of every physician executive gives PSNs an edge in being sensitive to these issues. That closeness to the patient experience is so important, and we distance ourselves from it at our peril.

By being able to pick and choose resources depending upon the special characteristics of a case, a network will be able to supply this customization. This is a tall order for an HSN. More than anything, it demands thinking outside the box. It means accessing different vendors at different times. It may demand reaching past customary providers to find one that is able to perform a particular service. This flexibility is not easy for anyone. But the flattened structure of a PSN gives it an edge in being able to step into the breach if the conditions require it. It perhaps will lead some hospitals as part of their strategic planning to step back from network formation altogether. This conflicts with the traditional philosophy that the hospital tries to be all things to all people, an idea that has driven much HSN development. It would, however, open a valuable niche for the hospital by allowing it to concentrate its resources on delivering the services that are truly needed in the community. By eliminating the drain that setting up and maintaining a network represents, hospitals may be positioning themselves far more effectively.

Many healthcare organizations, including hospitals, insurers, and HMOs, went on a buying spree in the 1980s in an attempt to diversify. This was primarily a "survivor" strategy; by so doing, each hoped to hedge against the uncertainty in healthcare. Now that the late 1990s have given some clarity to the direction of the industry, many are now shedding these acquisitions. They are distractions from what the organization's core purpose really is. Why does a hospital need to own a garage? Why does an HMO need to own a life insurance company? Likewise, it may well be time for hospitals to move away from their network development and decide how to make themselves most attractive to the networks that will survive. I believe the winners will be PSNs. But hospitals can be winners as well by grasping the reality of the new medical landscape and getting there first. This may not be the message hospital executives want to hear. The PHOs that popped up in the early 1990s were seen as a way of creating HSNs, although it may have been unspoken. The premier hospital system of the future (and that future is only a few years away) will work harmoniously with payors and networks as vendors but will not waste money trying to compete with them. This will actually make them stronger in the long run, as has happened frequently in other industries.

Refocusing, like all change, is painful. It is not easy to walk away from a cherished strategy. But it should be evident that network formation on

In 1996 the division of AT&T into three companies was traumatic. A venerable institution with the most widely held public stock in the United States was dismantling itself. Ma Bell was setting afloat the famous Bell Labs (reborn as Lucent Technologies) that had produced so many Nobel Laureates. Yet it was necessary for AT&T to focus on its core business of providing telecommunications in the digital age. Although the short-term results have been rocky for AT&T, it is far better situated now to compete against its powerful rivals. And the spin-offs, Lucent and NCR, have seen their performances improve dramatically as well.

the hospital side is flawed. Many hospitals will obviously continue to pursue it, and in some unique areas (rural or sparsely populated markets) it still may make some sense. For the vast majority of the 6,000 hospitals that remain in the United States, however, it is a losing proposition.

Strategic Planning for the PSN

The strategic planning process for a PSN will necessarily be different than that for a hospital if only because the hospital is a going concern. The PSN is often a vision held by a few physicians who see the need and the opportunity. Bringing something out of nothing is a true challenge, yet it can be very fulfilling. It is also important to remember the pitfall described by Steven Covey that reflects on this process: "Things are created twice; there is a mental, or first creation, and a physical, or second creation." (Most business failures begin in the first [Filley 1978] through lack of a business plan, lack of a vision, undercapitalization, etc.) A careful, detailed process is necessary. Rather than rehash some of the excellent guides to strategic planning available in any business school library, it is more useful to share some key discussion points that will provoke the kind of deep analysis this job must have.

First and foremost is the question posed earlier: Why do we want to put together a PSN? The kind of vision that will sustain this enterprise must spring from a desire to practice medicine in a better way and a proactive approach to healthcare trends. This may take a fair amount of philosophical wrestling before the leadership team can come together. But it must be done—it is that simple and that important. Having decided to be a "change leader" versus a follower or, even worse, a change-resister, a series of development questions should be considered. The more flesh that can be added by the planning process, the higher the probability of success as one moves to Covey's "second creation."

1. Who are our customers?

Customer focus is rightly the first item on the agenda. This will define the basic tenor of the PSN. Who do we want to reach? Where are they? Are we correct in targeting this market?

2. What do they need and expect?

This links back to the discussion of the patient's idea of what "seamless" means. It is different for the patient than for the network; each has different pressures, needs, constraints, etc. Therefore, once the customers are identified, the next logical step is to stand in their shoes and understand what will satisfy them. What does good service mean to the customer? What events would make them more likely to choose us?

3. What can we do to meet and exceed those needs?

Are these expectations achievable for us? Be very careful of not setting yourself up to fail. Some expectations may well be beyond your resources or ability. It is best to know this up front. This requires an honest self-assessment.

It is also good to have "stretch goals." The current status of the network may not be sufficient to serve these customers. What then can be done, with some effort and in a reasonable time frame, to be able to perform at that level? For example, there are no oncologists. How then can oncologic services be obtained by the effective date?

4. How can we monitor our progress?

This is the issue of accountability, which is one of the cornerstones of managed care. Health plans are accountable to employers for meeting their financial goals and servicing the contract. Physicians must be accountable for measurable, objective, reasonable outcomes. This is a dramatic change from the past when the measure of success was the discharge of a live (versus dead) patient from the hospital. Whether that person ever regained full functioning, went back to work, or even survived for more than a few weeks was not part of the definition of successful care (hence the old adage: "the operation was a success, but the patient died"). Any network—especially one composed of the primary providers of care, doctors—must be able to demonstrate longitudinal outcomes. Ideally, those should be *good* outcomes, too. The ability to conform to HEDIS and Foundation for Accountability (FACCT) measures will be the ticket of admission for such networks. Any that cannot do it will not be able to make the short list of candidates. Thus, attention to tracking outcomes, analyzing them, and feeding them back to the physicians must become routine. In any new PSN, this should start on day one, with the first patient.

Whenever data profiling is presented to physicians, there are two problems that immediately are raised. First, are the data credible? Second, that is all well and good but my patients are sicker. To achieve that crucial buy-in of the network physicians, both of these concerns must be satisfactorily explained. Only then can the discussion move forward as to how to use this profiling to change behavior, improve care, and close the loop on accountability. The planning for data collection, analysis, and reporting must take this into account.

5. What value do we bring to the market?

This is a tough question. It can only be answered once the group is able to assess the marketplace objectively. This means understanding the overcapacity and misutilization of medical resources, including hospitals, procedures, etc. It also means taking a walk in the shoes of the purchasers and consumers. While all providers feel they deliver unique value, this is not what the customers perceive. What is really the difference between St. John's and community hospitals? Between Drs. Smith and Jones? We must also keep in mind the Value Equation:

$$\textbf{High Quality Care + High Quality Service +}$$
$$\textbf{Reasonable Price = Value}$$

We can reorder or amend these factors, but the basic premise remains the same (see Table 3.4). Value is a combination of various elements that must all be delivered for value to exist. A common misunderstanding of medical providers is that service and price are not important to the patient. It is a bedrock of medical mythology that patients will follow their doctors wherever they go and will pay a premium for the care they receive in order to remain with their doctor. This perception was perhaps reality in the past when costs in general were low and insurance and reimbursement were not issues. It also reflects what I have referred to as the cottage industry mind-set of traditional medicine. But just as the corner pharmacy has been jolted by the large chains that offer better prices and discounts on very expensive medications, physicians and hospitals in the 1990s have priced themselves out of this quaint scenario of patients trooping across town, wallets in hand, to patronize a cherished provider. Value will bring those patients in, not nostalgia or misguided loyalties. But this opens up a wonderful opportunity for the networks that take the time to study carefully the new realities and learn what vacuums exist. Then the decision becomes how best to fill those vacuums.

6. What value do we convey to our customers?

This is a corollary to identifying the value you are bringing to the table. Hopefully, most providers will discover that they are positioned to actually improve the health of the people they serve. (Remember, most do not, and some actually diminish the health of their customers.) The question becomes how best to convey this message. The significance of the value brought to the market is the salient point: How does this value-added care differentiate your network from all the others? Is the result so

Table 3.4   More Value Diagrams

Various ways to depict the interaction between the elements of value:
1. **Value = Quality/Cost**
     where: Quality = Positive Change in Functional Status + Customer Service
     and: Cost = Total Cost of Care and Illness
                         (i.e., entire course of illness episode is calculated)
2. **Value = f (Quality, Cost, Access)**
     Where each factor is independently defined and exists in a nonlinear relationship
     with the others. Value becomes a function of the interaction among these factors.

A variety of such equations can be postulated to explain the relationships among the
elements of value that satisfy the requirements of a given clinical situation or medical
context. The goal should be to design an equation that is meaningful and answers the
question of what needs to be monitored and improved to provide value as perceived
by the customer.

meaningful that the customer can appreciate a significant improvement
in outcomes? Answering these questions will lead the PSN into a quality
improvement cycle as it seeks to make its results clinically important. For
example, a network may perform a particular function or service well, but
it is not refined or widespread enough for an employer to see the benefits
accrue to the bulk of the employees. A quality improvement approach
would be to rework this function, improving it in multiple small ways over
time to raise the value of it steadily. Business and industry understand
quality better than we do in medicine. Pareto charts, CQI teams, etc.,
have been innovations brought to the medical field from the experience
of industrial engineers. Its implementation within the framework of the
network, and its strong support by leadership, is a signal to customers
that the network believes in quality and value differentiation.

7. How do we measurably improve the practices and careers of our physicians?

So much time is spent discussing how the network serves customers that
it is easy to forget that a network, particularly a PSN, must also serve
the physicians who are part of it. They are, in effect, internal customers.
Contrary to those who see the managed care experience as closing out
the chances for individual professional development and growth, I see it
as an extraordinary opportunity to improve the way we practice. For the
first time in several generations, we are being given the tools to markedly
improve the health of the people we serve. This is in contrast to delivering
"sick" care, which focuses on episodes of illness but really does nothing
to prevent them or improve health status. Not since the great public

health triumphs of the early 1900s—the reduction of TB rates and the elimination of rickets and most fatal childhood diseases—have American physicians been present at such advances in health knowledge. These medical successes were based on the benefits brought to large numbers of people, populations in fact, versus a reduction in illness on a case-by-case basis. Likewise, we are finally inventing the tools and gaining the knowledge base that will allow us to make similar advances for our populations. It is exciting to realize we may begin to reduce some of the persistent diseases such as diabetes and breast cancer by approaching them in this manner.

This is part of the renaissance in medical practice that I have been suggesting is a result of the managed care revolution. This will result in a dramatic increase in the satisfaction and rewards of most practitioners. How can this be since the rap against managed care is its fixation with reducing physicians' salaries? Actually, what managed care is designed to do is decrease variation, inappropriate care, and unnecessary treatments. It is also designed to foster innovation and new technologies that can be shown to be medically sound and that address the issues of improving the health of populations. It is probable that most physicians will continue to see their incomes rise for the foreseeable future. Multiple surveys confirm that despite reductions in Medicare reimbursements and the spread of capitation, physicians' incomes rose 4.4 percent in 1995 and 7 percent in 1996, easily beating the rise in the cost of living (*Modern Healthcare* 1997). For the 14 largest specialties, all recorded increases, even in general surgery and anesthesiology (considered two of the most crowded and least desirable specialties to payors). This will continue as payors direct even more of their members into networks as the total number of health plans increases (Lippman 1997).

The message is that physicians can expect to do well economically even as managed care expands. They can also expect to be part of a new wave of medical progress as we seek to improve the health status of huge groups of people, not just one at a time. The challenge for the PSN then is to design a new pattern of care delivery that makes sense for the doctors as well as the patients. How does the network serve the physicians? What does it do to increase their satisfaction in practicing medicine? Are there innovative ways to bring *value*—separate from just money—back to the medical practices? As physicians are more sought after by expanding networks, they will become more selective in who they join. The PSN that can pass value back to the practitioner will be at an advantage in recruiting and retaining high-quality staff. That staff will then be more supportive of the PSN's objectives and will probably do a better job for the patients, especially on the service end. The result is a mutually reinforcing positive cycle that spreads the value to all participants: physician, network, patient, health plan, employer.

8. What is the business plan, in one-, three-, and five-year increments?

Both short- and long-term strategies are required. It is amusing to see a start-up HMO with 2,000 members detailing its employee pension plan after 30 years of service. It is frightening to see a PSN receive a large capitation check, whose officers then lease expensive offices and cars, only to go bankrupt in 18 months when huge incurred-but-not-received (IBNR) claims hit the system. The point is the absolute need for planning. Being in business demands that a timeline and goals be established that will serve as markers of progress or deviation. Any participating physician should be leery of joining a network that does not fully understand this, yet is able to lay out plans for the future. Further, such plans should make sense and be grounded in reality. What is a reasonable expectation of market share in a year? Are the projected capitation numbers realistic? What is the basis for anticipating the growth in contracts? What contingencies have been made for problems implementing the new information system?

9. How do we establish the sources of capital required to be successful?

Capital is a major hurdle for the PSN, unlike the HSN that can draw from a hospital's kitty. Extreme due diligence is necessary to avoid either undercapitalization or selling to a large entity that may have a different plan for the PSN. The Coastal example given earlier is sobering. So much money was spent on acquiring practices that those groups that did sell were not supported later.

10. What infrastructure will support the above objectives?

A fatal flaw in physicians' thinking is believing that the one-on-one interaction with the patient is sufficient to carry an organization. While this relationship is the heart of a medical delivery system, there must be the business components that make a network, versus a small practice, viable. Information systems is probably the most critical component, followed closely by good financial controls and systems. There are in fact a host of support services that are indispensable to any functioning managed care group.

Building the infrastructure is expensive. This is no time to be cheap. It's also good strategy to figure out how to position the network at the *front* of the pack. Being in the middle is not good enough. Payors will seek out those providers who are innovative and thinking outside the box; this point has already been stressed. Maximum segment differentiation is the key to outdistancing competitors. This does not mean simply throwing money at problems. A variety of knotty issues can be solved for next to nothing: relationships among the network members, interactions with important vendors, the character of the delivery system, the philosophy of the entire organization. These factors are far more significant than having a top-of-the-line computer system (that no one may know how to run). Once again, we find ourselves coming back to the basics: leadership, people skills, knowledge of the market, and players. It means intensive research into the intricacies of the business and making the best possible decisions with the tools and information available. *In medicine we sell service.* Do not become confused over this point. We use technology but it is the "soft" aspects of the medical practice that make a winner or an also-ran.

Potential Minefields

The road to the future is littered with broken networks. A multitude of dangers exists. It is impossible to foresee them all, but some obvious ones can be discussed.

"Providers as payors" is the most deadly. The belief that insurers are paid excessively to do mindless bureaucratic paperwork is rampant in the medical community. It overlooks the complexity of the insurance function and the difficulty many companies have in making money. A number of larger managed care organizations saw a downturn in 1997 despite the impression in the media that MCOs are making huge profits at the expense of consumers (*Wall Street Journal* 1997c). Unfortunately, this belief does not seem to lose its currency with time. The development questions detailed earlier would seem to settle this question and illustrate the potential disasters awaiting the unprepared who venture into the payor arena. But it is worth pointing out four additional areas that PSNs tend to ignore.

1. Underwriting is extremely difficult. State and federal regulations often prevent underwriting, virtually guaranteeing losses on some groups. A PSN-HMO would be forced to take high-risk groups that it may not be equipped to predict costs for accurately, leading to dire financial implications.

2. It is not possible to justify high rates to employers by simply saying "your employees are sicker." A PSN-HMO would have to prove this through extensive case-severity adjustment. Even when it is

able to demonstrate higher morbidity necessitating higher premiums, it could lose the contract to a larger health plan that has deeper pockets (and may see this particular contract as a loss leader).

3. Unrealistic expectations are common in organizations that stray from their core competency. Remember that a theme of this book is that the key to success in the new environment is to focus on core competencies and run with them. I once sat in on a presentation by a new health plan being sponsored by a large academic faculty practice that saw a niche for an HMO linked to the academic medical center. The prime strategy for the new plan was to offer a lower rate based on an administrative fee that would be 25 percent below all other competitors. When asked how this would be effected (when the other plans with more experience and resources could not offer lower rates), the answer was: "We will be more efficient." This type of simplistic (if not naive) approach is guaranteed to backfire, as in fact it did for this plan.

4. PSNs tend to function as physicians first. This is generally fine; I believe it is the strength of the PSN versus other network models. But it leads the physicians to forget they need more *members* than patients (Kongstvedt 1996). Therefore, they must market beyond their patient panels to avoid adverse selection (and the PSN must fully understand what adverse selection is). This entails looking at the community from a population instead of an individual perspective. The physicians must tolerate having a panel for which they are accountable but of which they treat only some of the patients. Likewise, enrolling large numbers of sick patients, even though it bolsters panels, can easily drive up costs far beyond premium revenue.

Administrative costs are often disdained by physicians, although better understood by healthcare executives. For-profit health plans have been mercilessly criticized for having rock-bottom costs and too much profit. Not-for-profit plans, especially the Blues, may experience the exact opposite. Regardless, the PSN needs to budget administrative costs realistically and understand its importance. A shortcut to higher reimbursement for participating practitioners cannot be found by arbitrarily gutting administrative expenses. Like everything in the healthcare arena, it is also a double-edged sword. Uncontrolled costs can easily eat a plan alive.

What Does This Mean for the Hospital?

I started this book by saying that everything you know is wrong. One traditional hallmark of American medicine has been the close links between doctor and hospital. These links are becoming less relevant. The movement away from hospital as center of the delivery system is well under way. Fewer physicians want or even need hospital privileges. More specialists are practicing in fields that will never admit a patient, such as dermatology. (When I was a resident at the University of Chicago, we had an entire inpatient floor for dermatology patients.) Healthcare executives will be obliged to reexamine the role of their institutions with respect to this shift in emphasis. As payors continue to push down inpatient costs, and PSNs accelerate in their development, the natural outcome of this movement will be to reconfigure the hospital as a specialized vendor occupying a certain niche.

Technology has moved out of the exclusive domain of the hospital, and the trend for the future is to promote primary care instead of high-resource-based specialty care. The hospitals that align themselves as the preferred providers for the more dynamic PSNs will be on the inside track to capture as much business as possible. Marketing to both clients—the PSN and the payor—will be the best way to gain control of this segment of the market. At the same time, PSNs will become more discerning as they become more sophisticated and realize there are multiple possibilities for directing their patients. As with most of the new paradigms in health, it is an unsettling change, yet also a dramatic opportunity for growth and redefining the mission of the hospital in the medical delivery system.

References

Carlson, R. P. 1997. "What Lies Ahead? Where Are We Going?" *Physician Executive* 23 (5): 14–26.

Cincinnati Enquirer. 1997. 31 July: 6.

Covey, S. 1990. *The 7 Habits of Highly Effective People.* New York: Simon & Schuster.

Deogun, N. 1996. "Bitter Medicine: Networks of Doctors Develop Big Problems." *Wall Street Journal* 26 September: A1.

Filley, A. C. 1978. *The Complete Manager.* Middleton, WI: Green Briar Press.

Kaiser Family Foundation. 1997. Press release. 21 August.

Kassirer, J. P. 1997. "Managing Managed Care's Tarnished Image." *New England Journal of Medicine* 337: 338–39.

Kuttner, R. 1997. "Physician-Operated Networks and the New Anti-Trust Guidelines." *New England Journal of Medicine* 336 (5): 386–89.

Kongstvedt, P. 1996. *The Managed Care Handbook.* Gaithersburg, MD: Aspen Publishers.

Lippmann, H. 1997. "Another Health Cost Explosion: It Is Not Inevitable." *Business and Health* March: 32.

Marr, T. J., and D. K. Risner. 1997. "When Is a Physician Network a Group?" *Partners Integration Advisor* 5 (4): 1.

Medical Economics. 1997. "Roping Down Managed Care." July: 46–50.

Medical Interface. 1996. January: 6.

Modern Healthcare. 1997 Physicians Compensation Report.

New York Times. 1997. "A Hospital Chain's Brass Knuckles, and the Backlash." 11 May.

Pallarito, K. 1996. "Babes in Managed-Care Land: Provider-Sponsored Networks Are Stepping Cautiously into Risk Contracting." *Modern Healthcare* 18 November: 32–40.

Peters, T. 1988. *Thriving on Chaos*. New York: Harper Collins.

van Amerongen, D. 1996. "Survey of CEOs and Medical Staff Presidents in the Atlantic Health Alliance." Management application paper, University of Wisconsin Department of Administrative Medicine.

Wall Street Journal. 1997a. 24 April: B1.

———. 1997b. 29 July: A1.

———. 1997c. "HMO's Woes Reflect Conflicting Demands of American Public." 22 December: A1.

ACADEMIC MEDICAL CENTERS
AND NETWORK STRATEGY

"For academic medical centers, coming to the table [with managed care organizations] with outcomes data is a particularly difficult dilemma. Clinical chiefs in AMCs truly believe that they deliver Cadillacs at Cadillac prices. When the CEO pushes them for evidence, they are met with incredulous looks or worse. The tripartite mission of AMCs— teaching, research and patient care—may not always promote the best outcomes, certainly not at the best price."

—David B. Nash, M.D., 1996

"We have trained those who are strangling us."

—Academic physician referring to community physicians, 1997

ACADEMIC MEDICAL centers (AMCs) hold a unique position in medicine. They are the centers of research that have powered the phenomenal transformation of medical science in this country. Even though few Americans ever have cause to use one, AMCs have a disproportionate impact on medicine and the politics of medical care delivery. The Medicare system was designed in large part to provide AMCs with a hidden subsidy to enable them to carry out their teaching and research missions (Yohalem and Brecher 1974). This fostered a dramatic growth in the late 1960s and throughout the 1970s in the size and number of residency programs (*Journal of the American Medical Association* 1973). As a result, most physicians, and virtually every specialist, have trained in one. The lore of the AMC continues to this day as new advances in medical care or a new "life-saving" procedure is announced in the lay press with the local AMC as backdrop to the visual.

Yet the future has become cloudy for AMCs. The upheavals in medical delivery have hardly bypassed them. In 1994, 30 of 126 AMCs had drops in revenue, versus only 18 in 1991 (Washington Press 1995). The average cost per case at AMCs in 1994 was $8,822 versus $5,020 for nonteaching hospitals. All AMCs face high fixed costs that remain regardless of the volume of patients (*Physicians Financial News* 1995). Since such differences are not lost on payors or other customers of the AMCs, the need to address them is acute.

Central Problems for AMCs

The dilemma for AMCs is the result of the restructuring of the medical marketplace. Previously, the AMC produced a series of goods for which there seemed to be unlimited demand. Research and teaching were always paired with patient care to create a triumvirate of missions that AMCs were established to deliver. It is an ongoing debate as to the relevant importance of each of these elements. It is also at the core of the conflict between the AMC and the community hospital, as well as between the academic physician and the community practitioner. It has led to an uncomfortable distance between the two groups, one that has resulted in competitive disadvantages for the AMCs. As primary care has become the cornerstone of managed care philosophy, it is obvious that many AMCs are out of the loop. Recent studies have shown a failure of AMCs to acknowledge primary care's increasingly important role, or to even present primary care in a positive light to the medical students and residents in training (Block et al. 1996). This has put the AMC somewhat out of step with most healthcare analysts. Employers and insurers see coordination of care and a holistic approach to the patients as a most positive trend for the future. At the same time, generalists are being disparaged, ambulatory care is not considered a priority, and few of the most visible AMCs are even offering primary care training (Katz 1997). This schism has yet to be confronted by academic medicine. Until it is, it will continue to be a source of friction with the broader community.

Research and teaching will continue to be important functions of the AMC. However, the relative value with respect to patient care must be more clearly defined. The AMC of the 1970s was predicated on a vision of research and education as ends unto themselves. In an era of limited resources, this is no longer realistic. Just as a physician must define his or her core competency, AMCs must do the same. Pure research may well be a luxury that few AMCs can afford. Or, if they do choose to pursue it, they must be prepared to fund it through mechanisms other than cross-subsidization from third-party payors.

A different way to consider this is the concept of public and private goods. Private goods are sold to customers and include medical care, education, and some research (Blumenthal and Meyer 1996). Public goods are services for which there is no private market but that are valuable to society. This would include care of indigent groups, basic medical research, and training health professionals. Each class of good has been a rich source of revenue for AMCs in the past. AMCs have usually charged anywhere from 15 percent to 35 percent more than comparable institutions for their services. The premise has been that the (presumably) better care and the prestige of being at the AMC justified the higher charges (Golembesky 1995). But the competitive advantage of having an AMC in the network has been difficult to prove. A recent analysis of AMC contracting indicated the value payors place on AMCs is in the 3 percent to 5 percent range, a significant shortfall from the rates being charged. This discrepancy in value perception illustrates the crisis AMCs are facing in the medical landscape.

Just as the worth of the private goods AMCs produce is under pressure, so is that of the public goods. AMCs certainly fulfill an important role in delivering care to indigent groups and underserved populations. With the growth of Medicare and Medicaid, these activities have become increasingly central to the operations of most AMCs. The contribution of government subsidies to AMCs is substantial. As these programs are scaled back over the next few years, AMCs will be hit hard on the bottom line. This becomes another significant source of revenue shortfall.

Competition from other providers has become a major concern for AMCs. This was not so in the past when the AMC was the sole owner of high technology and specialty services. Until relatively recently, it was impossible to receive sophisticated care except at the AMC. As the number of subspecialists mushroomed, they needed to find places to practice once the AMCs had filled their departmental staffs. Medical technology vendors were only too happy to start calling on well-heeled community hospitals seeking to develop new specialty programs. Consequently, today we find more advanced infertility programs outside the AMCs than inside. Almost any high-tech diagnostic procedure can be obtained outside the AMC. For the insurer, this has been a welcome shift. These services can now be found more conveniently for patients and less expensively for payors. Burdened by high overhead and nonmedical costs, AMCs are at an increasing disadvantage as well on customer service and convenience issues. AMCs have yet to demonstrate convincingly that they are capable of cost-effective care and lower utilization. They are also unable to show that the quality of care rendered is so superior to other hospitals, except for rare and highly complex diseases, as to warrant higher charges. Immune from competition for most of this century, AMCs are facing competitive pressures as never before.

Much of this situation is not the fault of the AMC. As an institution, the AMC has done a credible job. The problem has been the inability of the AMC to recognize the new trends in healthcare and to respond appropriately or promptly. The huge bureaucracy that exists within most AMCs remains a barrier to the kind of flexibility that permits speedy change. The reclusive nature of many academic physicians has not helped. And the perception of most lay people of the AMC has not been positive. It has certainly not been what academic leaders think it should be. An Association of American Medical Colleges survey reveals most Americans do not connect AMCs to quality care because they do not understand what such institutions do (*Modern Healthcare* 1997b). As the report stated, "Americans believe this country's medical education, care and research are among the finest in the world. They do not, however, connect the terms 'academic medical center' or 'academic medicine' with these highly valued outcomes."

This, then, is the challenge for AMCs for the near future: the central problems of loss of guaranteed revenue sources, higher-than-market charges, a mission that is not valued by payors, antagonism toward primary care, and outcomes that are not appreciated by the public. AMCs are becoming more innovative and aggressive in their approaches to these problems. Network formation has been a key strategy for many. It is a way for the AMC to transform its organization, reach out to the community, and prepare for the "new" AMC of the next century. It will be a rather different looking animal than the AMC of the past.

Network Strategy Within the Academic Context

AMCs must deal with a variety of problems, and do so simultaneously to remain viable. They must address the central problems listed above, while they position themselves to be more attractive to payors. They must satisfy the needs of primary care physicians and give them reasons to form linkages with the AMC. Before any real progress on these fronts can be made, however, the AMC must resolve some important internal conflicts.

First, the AMC must understand what a network is and what it can and cannot do. PHOs have shown the fallacy of slapping together a "network" from several medical staffs and expecting this to translate into meaningful patient flow or new patterns of care. As discussed in Chapter

2, if this is a knee-jerk reaction to a market change, it is guaranteed to fail. There must be an acceptance of the reality ("gain power by accepting reality"). Only by "moving past the debate" and concentrating on how to deal with the new paradigm can progress be made.

A network means forming ties to groups and organizations outside the institution. For many AMCs, this has never been done before. Establishing a network entails bringing external participants into the AMC fold. Opening up the medical staff, changing referral processes, etc., can be traumatic if the AMC has resisted this in the past. Yet it must be done if the network is to become functional. AMCs and their medical faculties need to know the barriers that have been erected over time and that keep most primary care physicians (PCPs) out of the academic setting. Some of the barriers are unintentional and result from the difficulty in working with a large, ponderous organization, especially since few AMCs have ever been concerned about physician satisfaction or customer service. Some barriers are definitely intentional, such as the absence of family medicine physicians on staff. The refusal to establish departments of family practice is often no accident. In today's environment, such discrimination makes little sense and only serves to isolate the AMC from the mainstream. Given the popularity of PCPs among payors, the government, and patients, the onus is on the AMC to resolve this internal conflict and reach out to community practitioners. Until this is done in a sincere fashion, and in a manner designed to bring value to the larger lay public as well as the AMC, it will be almost impossible to set up a network that can accomplish what it must.

Another internal conflict that must be settled is the factionalism between various specialties and departments. This accompanies the realignment of the AMC's mission as being externally focused instead of purely internally focused. Many AMCs have grown into small feudal baronies, with departments jealously guarding their fiefs from each other. Scant attention was usually paid to events outside the halls of the AMC. Hence the most important department politically in an AMC, often with the power of life or death over major projects, was one that had minimal contact with the "outside world." I am always intrigued to see the Departments of Pathology or Anesthesiology wield tremendous influence within an AMC, even though these departments never generate a single dollar of revenue independently. Indeed, many of their departmental members could not exist outside of the academic facility. As more and more care moves into the ambulatory center, such situations make less and less sense. It is these departments, however, that are most threatened by managed care. Not only are they unable to function directly as managed care providers, but as the hospital utilization declines, so does the need for their skills. AMCs must make some very difficult choices in how to structure the decision-making processes going forward. It may require breaking down these power structures if an option like network formation is to be implemented. Fiefdoms are not compatible with new patterns of care that use whatever service or resource is necessary for a given patient. Recall from Chapter 3 Tom Peter's example of the specialty team that comes together for a high-intensity project, then disbands.

The allocation of capital is always contentious. In an AMC, the furor is frequently magnified by the three missions of the AMC: teaching, research, and patient care. Who gets the larger piece of the pie? Should all the pieces be of equal size? Network development and restructuring of the AMC both occur at the same time. A network cannot be grafted onto an AMC, with the rest of the system untouched. The lack of success of HSNs shows this, as well as the lack of acceptance of this business model by payors. Just as demolishing the Berlin Wall swept aside the old hierarchies in East Germany, the destruction of the barriers preventing network formation will also shake up the AMC. It will also require that significant dollars be allocated to make this happen. To procure this capital, money may well need to be diverted from other areas, including research and education. Projects such as hospital expansion may need to be shelved, both to allot capital to networks and to avoid creating debt that will hamper new initiatives in the future. This was the trap AMCs in Philadelphia fell into.

> Despite managed care penetration of 32 percent in the Philadelphia market, AMCs there have not undertaken significant efforts to reduce overcapacity and overbedding (*Modern Healthcare* 1997c). They have rapidly built "networks" but these have not led to any profound restructuring. Duplication and excessive overhead are still rampant, with 3.85 beds per 1,000 population (versus 2.26 per 1,000 in Sacramento, a similarly mature managed care market). As a consequence, extreme price competition has broken out, benefiting carriers but hammering the AMCs. Moody's Investor Services has downgraded the bonds of all four AMCs and stated to potential investors "the worst is yet to come."

The degenerating situation in Philadelphia illustrates the plight facing many AMCs. Blinded by their prestigious histories, the AMCs there were unable or unwilling to address forcefully the internal conflicts that must be resolved to proceed to building functional networks and coupling them with necessary structural change.

Models of AMC Network Strategy

There is a plethora of ways to configure a network centered on an AMC. The path to success must include the elements discussed above. The desire to take a stand and to accept change must be legitimate. If the AMC can get past these hurdles, quite a range of options is possible. The pitfall is to be so enamored of past glories that the need to get moving is not seen as imperative. The danger for AMCs, as with politicians, is to start believing one's own press clippings.

Presented briefly below are a few of those options. It can be plainly seen that they are variations on the themes put forth for HSNs. Each must be modified to meet the unique characteristics of the individual AMC. This involves taking into account a variety of dimensions not even on the radar screen for a typical hospital system, such as having adequate patient volumes to satisfy clinical teaching and research programs. Others are almost identical to problems confronting any hospital: decreasing admissions, lower reimbursement, excess capacity, and so forth.

Option 1: Leverage the AMC medical staff into an HSN that seeks to incorporate community physicians

This strategy is essentially creating an AMC HSN. It has several distinctive challenges over other HSN formation. First, there is the entire issue of "town versus gown," that is, the academic/community physician conflict. Culturally this clash can be quite dramatic. Each group feels the other is deficient in several necessary areas and that working together may well drag both down instead of up. Several examples will illustrate.

- For one AMC, setting up a network meant opening up the medical staff and faculty to the local physicians. For the faculty members, this was a sticking point. The department chairs did not believe, and said as much, that anyone not already on the medical staff was qualified to join.
- The work ethic of the two groups can conflict because of the different priorities of each. AMC faculty are not used to seeing patients more than a few sessions per week, and only a few patients per session. (This attitude is responsible for the low productivity of many staff model HMO physicians who come to the health plan straight out of residency. Such doctors make up a large portion of many staff models and prevent the HMOs from realizing their full potential.) Conversely, many private practitioners have an almost endless ability to expand office hours to accommodate demand, especially for fee-for-service patients.
- A major fear of some AMCs is the "franchising" of their name. Some see their name as proprietary to the point that they are unwilling to develop a network that would allow that name to be placed on sites that are not directly controlled by the institution (such as an affiliated practice). This is similar to the reluctance Apple Computer

has had to relinquish any control whatsoever of its brand name, even as Microsoft (which has no such reluctance) was driving Apple's market share into the low single digits.

All of these threats need to be dealt with and confronted directly. Assuming this is possible, then there is a real opportunity for successful network development by joining with local physicians. In many respects, such doctors are the on-site experts and bring value to the relationship with the AMC. A novel example is that of the Mayo Clinic's expansion into the northern Illinois area around Rockford. Recognizing that it draws almost 15,000 patients per year from that area, Mayo is constructing a network with a local hospital system and clinic (*Chicago Tribune* 1997).

Under the arrangement, Mayo physicians would travel to Rockford to see patients and deliver care, and provide continuing education for community physicians. Information systems support would also be given to the hospital to improve the links between them and their providers, as well as with Mayo itself. This accomplishes several purposes. It creates a regional plan for Mayo that is usually lacking in most AMC strategies. As employers look for regional or national care delivery systems, the attractiveness of a network bound to a limited geographic area decreases. One drawback of the traditional AMC is that it has existed as the hub of the wheel for local referral patterns. This is still the primary goal of most AMCs and for good reason: one needs to pay close attention to one's base. But to secure business beyond this limited field and to increase the likelihood of being included as a preferred provider or center of excellence, thought must be given to breaking out of this rut. Mayo is focused on being included in managed care contracts whenever possible. It will help avoid the marginalization that would occur if Mayo were unable to safeguard and expand its referral relationships. Mayo has also become comfortable with allowing community providers into the fold and sharing the Mayo name with them. It has evidently dealt successfully with the internal conflicts and is determined to move past them.

Option 2: Affiliate with area HSNs and/or PHOs

This is a simplistic approach, with low cost, low risk, and, predictably, low success rates. Simply to tag on to existing HSNs and present oneself as a "preferred provider" for the HSN (preferred in a generic, not a managed care, sense) is relatively meaningless. It seems attractive for an AMC that is reluctant to become fully engaged in redesign of its operations, but its lack of serious commitment will usually scuttle it. Two case studies are instructive.

- For one AMC in a highly developed managed care market, network formation consisted of announcing an alliance between it and seven area hospitals. The plan was for the various PHOs and the faculty of the academic center to come together under a joint board and develop new approaches to care for the region. While several of the hospitals were quite excited over this configuration, the problem was that no one bothered to tell the rank and file at the AMC. There was scant support for any sharing of time or expertise with the "partners." None of the internal conflicts had been addressed, much less resolved. Part of the issue was a failure of the AMC leadership, both administrative and medical, to properly convey a sense of urgency to the faculty that would justify undertaking this new direction in order to embrace change. There was no perception of a need to do anything different, hence no groundswell of support for any initiative that would disrupt the status quo. As a result of a deficit of physician leadership—a theme I continue to stress—$1 million in seed money from the AMC quickly disappeared without one patient visit to the academic hospital to show for it.

- For another AMC already developing its own HSN, the attempt to forge a relationship with several local HSNs was blunted by a failure to focus on a single strategy. At the same time this project was under way, the AMC was also entering into discussions with hospitals that competed with the first set of HSNs. The academic faculty, which again had not been brought in on the ground level and made a full participant in the planning, was confused and had not committed itself to any of the processes. At the end of the day, none of the talks bore fruit and the AMC HSN was left without any community links.

This points out another potential roadblock to AMC strategy. There must be an analysis done to determine whether the arrangements being proposed are realistic. Sitting in the academic center, it is deceptively easy to rationalize that barriers to plans will melt away. One can convince oneself that, yes, people will drive for long distances, and past other hospitals, to reach your facility. From the outside this looks much less likely.

Recently, one East Coast academic health system entered into an affiliation with a suburban hospital almost 50 miles away in an adjacent metropolitan area (and only four miles from two other well-known academic centers). On paper, this may appear as another affiliation to add to others, giving the impression of depth and breath of care delivery. Realistically, it is highly doubtful it will ever generate more than a handful of clinical interactions between the two geographically dispersed institutions (interactions that may have occurred anyway). The time and resources devoted to this project are unlikely ever to be recovered. It could also have some negative ramifications as the two AMCs feel slighted or offended by a joint venture happening in their backyard.

One last issue on this topic: embarking on poorly thought-out projects runs a risk not only of present failure but of future failure. The potential affiliates who find their time and resources wasted by the AMC are not going to be lining up to participate in another venture with it. By poisoning the well through unfocused and unrealistic initiatives, the AMC gains the worst kind of reputation—that of an organization that is unable to develop meaningful projects and see them through. The community providers are then almost forced into searching other, nonacademic alternatives as they try to stay competitive.

Option 3: Merge AMCs

Merging AMCs has great potential if done properly and with a steady eye on eliminating duplication and promoting efficiency. A good example is Partners Health Care System (PHCS) in Boston, consisting of Massachusetts General Hospital and Brigham and Women's Hospital (Blumenthal and Meyer 1996). PHCS is located in an advanced, stage III managed care marketplace, yet maintains an 81.5 percent occupancy rate. It has a war chest of perhaps billions of dollars, all the while it has 32 percent HMO patients and 10 percent Medicaid patients. PHCS leaders plan to close 700 of their 1,700 beds over the next five years, the equivalent of a large teaching hospital in itself. Their efforts to improve operations and eliminate redundancy stand in stark contrast to the Philadelphia case cited earlier. PHCS suggests that a merger can be an effective strategy if conflicts and problems are faced directly and resolved. Being competitive implies being able to make rapid, well-informed decisions, without the necessity of being bogged down in bureaucracy. PHCS has apparently achieved this end, while reducing the cost of care and maintaining a healthy financial surplus.

Option 4: Create a Specialty Network Anchored by an AMC

This is an innovative but risky method of network formation. It involves using the AMC and its faculty as the nucleus for a managed care product that will then be the vehicle to build the network of community providers. It has several interesting advantages. By using a high-profile name (that of the AMC), its entry into the market will be more easily accomplished than a routine startup. This name will also hopefully attract some skilled partners on the business and administrative sides. It also brings to discussions with local doctors two very important elements: patients and money. It does not necessarily demand that the academic medical staff open up to others, although this is desirable in the long run (and is, I believe, the only way to truly change attitudes and behaviors). It is also a way to reach reluctant employers who may have been loath to consider the AMC because of the significantly higher costs.

On the downside, this tactic carries much of the baggage that attaches to any provider-as-payor project. With an AMC, given the historic paucity of business acumen in academic medical circles, this is even riskier. Can the AMC faculty really deliver cost-effective care? Can a satisfactory care pattern between the AMC and area providers be established? Will the volumes be significant enough to catch their attention and preferentially use the network? And, can the network survive in the long term if the AMC faculty is unwilling to accept community doctors on staff and share decision making with them?

Beginning in the early 1980s, a number of AMCs developed their own HMOs. This is substantially different from a product since it was often just an extension of the AMC outpatient clinics and often designed to serve the medical center employees only. Some of these evolved into highly sophisticated networks that are thriving today, such as the Harvard Community Health Plan. The sticking point in any planning around an AMC-owned product or HMO is to be clear on the purpose. If there is an expectation that the product or HMO will replace volume lost to managed care or ambulatory services, one had better think again. Billi et al. analyzed the possibility of the University of Michigan's HMO, MCare, supporting the specialty services of the hospital at 1992 levels (Billi et al. 1995). Their conclusion was that over 1,000,000 enrollees would be required to do so, and that they would have to use the University of Michigan for the bulk of their care. This places this option far from the realm of the possible. We return to the fact that network formation must be grounded in reality to be effective. It is important to have a sense of history and tradition, for these are part of creating professionalism. But an AMC cannot use a reputation or even a regional monopoly as a proposed solution to increasing market competition.

One instance of a possible source of competitive advantage as well as focal segmentation for AMCs is to consider product formation based on one or more core competencies of the institution. A growing number of specialty networks are springing up at the same time specialists are starting to make the case that, for certain diseases, SCPs do a better job than PCPs (Jollis et al. 1996). Remember the theme of focusing on areas of competency: "know thy work and do it." In the same vein, AMCs that truly feel they can provide high-quality, cost-effective care for high-profile diseases may do well to market that fact in the form of a product tied to a network of specialists. A prototype for such a program may be the "Moore Options" HIV/AIDS program developed by Johns Hopkins (named after the Moore Clinic).

Moore Options

Moore Options is based on the changing nature of HIV and AIDS: seeing them as increasingly manageable chronic illnesses. Health plans and providers have the potential for keeping costs in line by implementing a coordinated approach to AIDS and HIV disease management programs (*Demand of Disease Management* 1997). The program at Hopkins provides services along a broad continuum from outpatient primary care to home healthcare and transportation. The program receives $2,160 per patient per month in capitation from several Medicaid managed care organizations. The results of the project have been impressive: lower length of stays for AIDS patients and lower costs per patient as the patient becomes sicker (as reflected by CD4 counts). (See Figure 4.1).

This experience has important implications for Johns Hopkins and, indeed, all AMCs. It is a demonstration to payors that high-quality, cost-effective care for chronic expensive diseases can be provided through a network of experienced specialists. It may well be for such patients that the best way to deliver their care is through a specialist-oriented system instead of the primary care physician who is not trained to deal with the enormous medical and social demands of this clientele. This is a powerful message because it creates a niche for AMC services and it offers an opportunity to prove that value exists in preferring the specialists' participation in managed care networks for these situations. The financial risk is borne by the network and the patient receives the best care available.

The product formation option has yet to reach its potential in that the relations with the community-based referral systems outside its immediate service area are weak (back to the "town vs. gown" issue), but it is a good template. It can serve as a model for other SCP networks focusing on difficult, high-intensity diseases. If these are the diseases, such as AIDS, that the government is willing to capitate or make other special reimbursement arrangement for, it could be quite lucrative for all involved. It would also serve as an entrée for other network initiatives between the AMC and the community.

There is another potential benefit to the AMC from taking the time to develop a specialty network. Such a program would help referring physicians by smoothing the path for their patients, particularly the ones with challenging medical problems. More important, as the popularity of open access options in managed care plans increases, it will position the AMC to receive this business. Many payors are reluctant to refer

Figure 4.1 Cost of Medical Care in HIV-Infected Patients

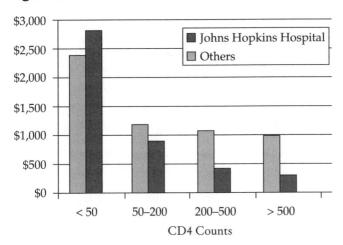

to AMCs; many feel the reputations are not justified by the level of quality of their services or the price. The discomfort academics feel as costs are reduced along with prices is a problem for payors who see this as simply creating value (recall the Value Equation in Chapter 3). But consumers have declared that they generally hate the HMO referral systems. In response, most plans are developing open access products that will allow members to see specialists within the network without prior authorization or a referral. For the AMC with a healthy volume of network providers, this could be a major boon. The hurdle is to get such a group up and running, which will entail convincing payors that the AMC is committed to managed care values. It may be a long while before people with chronic diseases such as diabetes or AIDS are assigned to SCPs as their primary providers, but those AMCs that begin working on this option will be there sooner rather than later.

Losing Strategies

Having presented a sampling of winning ideas, it is also necessary to consider those that are destined to fail. Again, it is important to step back and try to view the AMC dispassionately. What is its real position in the market? Do consumers feel the AMC is an indispensable clinical resource for the regions (especially if there are other AMCs locally)? What are the directions for Medicare and Medicaid patients in the area?

A host of potential losing strategies exist. A few are discussed below:

The effects of public sector health reform may well be as significant for some AMCs as what is occurring in the private sector. Many AMCs rely heavily on Medicaid patients to supply clinical as well as research volumes, not to mention providing revenue. State legislators may be drafting anti-managed care legislation by the truckload—more than 1,400 such bills were introduced in 1996 (Associated Press 1997)—but they are also pushing as much of their Medicaid populations into managed care as possible (admittedly a somewhat schizophrenic approach). The University of Texas is considering developing an HMO, since by 2000 all Texas Medicaid recipients will be required to be in a form of managed care (*Modern Healthcare* 1997a). In Tennessee, the state's radical shift of large groups of the uninsured into TennCare caused significant short-term disruptions at two of its four AMCs (Meyer and Blumenthal 1996). Both experienced large revenue shortfalls, the closure of some specialty services, adverse patient selection, loss of the patient volume needed to do clinical research in several areas, and a reduction in the number of training program positions. However, there may be a long-term silver lining to this upheaval. The rapid introduction of these patients into the AMC networks have sped up the integration of the networks with community-based services, accelerated clinical diversification, and improved the AMC's managed care business practices. All of these changes make the AMCs more aggressive, more knowledgeable, and more attractive to payors. They may well find themselves better positioned than before the TennCare experiment began.

Losing Strategy 1. Focusing on a segmented market with minimal potential for growth, or no impact on local care patterns

It is tempting to look for a niche to fill, even if that niche is not of great value. I have mentioned the importance of focal segmentation as a competitive advantage. By identifying recognizable groups that make up the market, one can then select one or several of them as a target market. But this only becomes an advantage if it is of demonstrable value to consumers, and has potential for generating volume and/or revenue. Some AMCs have tried to attract international patients, build Ritz-style rooms with concierge services, etc. These are glitzy and can merit an article in the local newspaper, but are of minimal worth. There will never be enough rich, sick foreigners to affect volumes or revenues in a sustainable, predictable (for budgeting purposes) manner. Efforts along these lines are fine as long as they do not detract from network and managed care initiatives as they frequently do. Such projects should also not be used as window dressing, that is, an excuse to fail to confront the internal conflicts that ultimately must be resolved. The danger is that these showpieces will not speak to the basic problems. AMCs continue to lose market share to community hospitals (Reuter and Gaskin 1997). This will only accelerate if attention is allowed to drift to nonproductive activities.

Losing Strategy 2. Creating "paper" alliances with local hospitals

This topic has already been broached. It is pointless to "sign up" affiliate members, call it a network, and expect any verifiable results to follow. Yet this is a common response by AMCs to competitive pressure from other hospital systems. The alliance framework has its positives and negatives (see Chapter 2). A major drawback for the prime sponsor (usually the AMC) is that the other participants (and I use this word loosely, since the commitment level is usually pretty low and participation is hard to document) are frequently pursuing multiple options at the same time. Those alternatives will occasionally even conflict with the "alliance," but if there is little commitment and few dollars at play, such conflicts are not corrected. The risk for the AMC in this setting is greater than that for the community networks. The AMC faculty may consider this a solution to the current crisis and therefore not proceed to do the groundwork required to become skilled managed care providers. Once the alliance fails to deliver, it will become a self-fulfilling prophesy, justifying the slow pace the AMC is taking to restructuring. This can then lead to Losing Strategy 3.

Losing Strategy 3. Raising the drawbridge

Out of frustration with the difficulties of internal restructuring, realigning departments, augmenting clinical services, etc., exhaustion may take over and then the AMC turns inward. This is also seen when a university board of trustees becomes mired in the question of the medical campus that used to be a cash cow and now is a sea of problems (a.k.a. a "cash pig"). Failure to face the external environment head-on can only lead to a neglect of the network formation process. The critical importance of the redirection of the AMC toward the community (and hence toward new partners like local providers, employers, payors, etc.) becomes submerged in the instinct to stick with what is familiar. The drawbridge goes up, the level of interaction with the outside goes down, and the window of opportunity to reshape the institution as a managed care provider closes.

Losing Strategy 4. Beginning network development without a primary care base

This encompasses not only an understanding of primary care but also having real, live primary care physicians on staff. The condescending attitudes of academic medicine toward primary care have previously been documented. Managed care has been built around the PCP-patient interaction, so having PCPs as key participants in the process from the start would seem axiomatic. Yet a surprising number of AMCs embark on ambitious network formation programs without securing their PCP base. As a consequence, they are not informed as to what primary care medicine needs in order to flourish. Cultural barriers must be reduced to allow the kinds of interactions with PCPs that will educate AMC leaders. Without the benefit of firsthand experience, the AMC will never be able to comprehend fully the market they are trying to enter or the service they are seeking to deliver. This lack of understanding can have dire effects and can make large sums of money disappear without a trace. And yet, for all their medical sophistication, large AMCs continue to plunge ahead blindly. One AMC in California began building and promoting its network (whose purpose was to become a community-based conduit to the AMC for local physicians) with only five PCPs on its faculty. This was topped by the Northeast AMC that spent several million dollars on Losing Strategies 1 and 2, but out of a staff of 1,200 physicians has only one board-certified family physician.

Do not mistake the praise given to Johns Hopkins for their specialist-based AIDS network as inferring that there is no need for the AMC to reach out to PCPs. The future for specialty networks is bright, and I believe many AMCs will profit substantially by developing them in certain areas. But this is, by definition, a niche strategy. It has no hope of capturing large volumes of business or of providing the kind of base on which any provider system needs to build. The bread and butter of any hospital of whatever type is unlikely to be delivered by a handful of specialty networks.

The AMC of the Twenty-First Century

Most AMCs are not likely to survive intact. There is no doubt that most, like those caught up in the TennCare tidal wave, will undergo gut-wrenching retrenchment. Programs will be downsized, even closed, as faculty are cut and beds shut down permanently. While most public AMCs will probably be supported to some degree by the states as a matter of local pride, many private AMCs may find it necessary to merge or sell out. While these transactions may or may not preserve the name of the AMC, its identity will be forever altered. But some AMCs will thrive and form the nucleus of a dynamic, progressive academic medical system. What will these AMCs look like, and what will distinguish them?

Above all, these will be the institutions that came to grips with change and made it work for them. They will have resolved the internal conflicts, cultural clashes between academia and the rest of the medical community, and confusion over the new direction of healthcare. They will have moved beyond these debates to engage in serious planning for providing those services. Their networks will reflect this. They will be modeled as links between the community and the AMC, with attention given to customer service, support for the primary care physicians, and a positive relationship with payors. These networks will obviously be heavily oriented toward specialty care, but there will be a strong primary care flavor to them in that PCPs will have had significant input to their design and implementation. This input is necessary to create a framework that is friendly to both patient and PCP, and to promote buy-in from the community. The AMC itself will be a reduced version of what it is today. It will have fewer beds, do fewer nondiagnostic procedures, and seek to avoid competition with local hospitals. It will be a much more complementary relationship than we now see.

As for the other two prongs of the academic mission, teaching and research, the network will play a crucial role in both. As mentioned, only a handful of diagnoses account for the bulk of medical admissions today. As ambulatory care continues to expand its horizons, this number will shrink further. For example, many oncology patients may never spend a single day as an inpatient. For a growing cohort of patients, diagnostics, biopsies, chemotherapy, and hospice care will be rendered outside the hospital. Hence, in order to teach medicine properly, the department chairman will have to make extensive use of the AMC network to get his or her residents out into the locations that are receiving the patient visits. This real-world experience will also prepare those residents more completely for "Life After Training" than in the past. Likewise, as more alternative research sites increase (as nonacademic contractors become involved in clinical trials [*Wall Street Journal* 1995]), different sources of funding and patients must be explored. Networks offer a viable way to access these resources and preserve at least some of the clinical research function. This activity will change, however. The need for outcomes research will only become more pressing with time. AMC networks will be uniquely qualified to perform these studies, for which many managed care organizations will pay well (*Wall Street Journal* 1997).

To traditionalists, these changes will seem to be heresy. The process of the AMC's mission will be radically different, but I believe its focus will remain the same: to supply society with highly trained physicians, perform valid research on the medical problems (including medical care delivery) that face us (and that society deems important), and take care of the sickest of our citizens. Networks will be a valuable tool in this transformation to the next generation of academic medicine.

References

Associated Press. 1997. "States Gear up to Battle to Regulate Managed Care." *www.ap.org:* 12 February.

Billi, J. E., C. E. Wise, E. A. Bills, and R. L. Mitchell. 1995. "Potential Effects of Managed Care on Specialty Practice at a University Medical Center." *New England Journal of Medicine* 333: 979–83.

Block, S. D., N. Clark-Chiarelli, A. S. Peters, and J. D. Singer. 1996. "Academia's Chilly Climate for Primary Care." *Journal of the American Medical Association* 276: 677–82.

Blumenthal, D., and G. S. Meyer. 1996. "Academic Health Centers in a Changing Environment." *Health Affairs* 15 (2): 200–15.

Chicago Tribune. 1997. "Mayo Clinic May Wake House Cell in Rockford." 27 June: C1.

Culbertson, R. A. 1995. *Comparison of Contracting Attributes in Maturing U.S. Health Care Markets.* Robert Wood Johnson Foundation.

Demand of Disease Management. 1997. "Specialist Drive Success of AIDS Disease Management." 3 (6): 81–86.

Golembesky, H. 1995. "New Market Forces Are Special Challenge to Academic Medical Center. *Physician Executive* 21: 18–22.

Jollis, J. G., E. R. Delong, E. D. Peterson, L. H. Muhlbaier, D. F. Fortin, R. M. Califf, and D. B. Mark. 1996. "Outcomes of Acute Myocardial Infarction According to the Specialty of Admitting Physician." *New England Journal of Medicine* 335: 1880–87.

Journal of the American Medical Association. 1973. "Graduate Medical Education: Annual Report on Graduate Medical Education in the United States." 226: 930–40.

Katz, L. A. 1997. "Where Will Managed Care Fit in Medical Education." *Journal of the American Medical Association* 277: 1038.

Meyer, G. S., and D. Blumenthal. 1996. "TennCare and Academic Medical Centers: The Lessons from Tennessee." *Journal of the American Medical Association* 276: 672–76.

Modern Healthcare. 1997a. "Regional News." 30 June: 86.

———. 1997b. "Identity Crisis: Teaching Hospitals Find They're Misunderstood." 13 January: 48–50.

———. 1997c. "Thumbs Down: Moody's Paint a Bleak Picture of Pa.'s Two Big Markets." 23 June: 28.

Physicians Financial News. 1995. "Surviving Managed Care Presents Challenge for Academic Medical Centers." 30 June: 1.

Reuter, J., and D. Gaskin, 1997. "Academic Health Centers in Competitive Markets." *Health Affairs* 16 (4): 242–52.

Wall Street Journal. 1995. "Change in Health Care Shakes up the Business of Drug Development." 28 March: A1.

———. 1997. "Business Bulletin." 22 January: A1.

Washington Press. 1995. "Pressure Mounts on Academic Medical Centers." 10 September: A6.

Yohalem, A. M., and C. M. Brecher. 1974. "The University Medical Center and the Metropolis: A Working Paper." In *The University Medical Center and the Metropolis,* edited by E. Ginzburg and A. M. Yohalm. New York: Josial Macy, Jr., Foundation.

5

THE PHYSICIAN-PAYOR AXIS

"The irony is that we Americans have the best medical care in human history. Period. The downside, we can't afford it."
—Leonard Shaetter, CEO, Blue Cross Blue Shield of California, 1995

THE VALUE and purpose of networks have hopefully become apparent during the course of this book. For most healthcare and physician executives, the issue is how to best construct a network that meets several functions. As shown in Table 5.1, each participant in the medical delivery process realizes value and positive outcomes. The table itself could be expanded to multiple pages to include all the possible ramifications of this analysis.

For the leader examining it and trying to divine the proper framework upon which to build the network, one important proviso should be remembered. After all is said and done, the heart of the healthcare system

Table 5.1 The Role of Networks

	Value	Outcome
Physician	Access to patients	Operational support; autonomy
Patient	Access to quality M.D.s and services	Quality care at affordable costs
Employer	Predictable expenses; satisfied, well-cared for employees	Higher employee productivity; reasonable healthcare costs
Health Plan	Able to offer quality, desirable products	Improved health measures for members

is the physician. Try as they may, insurance executives, Congress, and others have been unable to design a medical care process that does not ultimately rely on a doctor laying hands upon a patient. Even in China, home of the "Barefoot Doctor" and heavily dependent on nonphysician delivery models, the doctor is still the most important player, seeking to touch the distant patient through the intermediary of the lay assistant. We need to constantly remind ourselves of this fact so we can keep network formation in the proper context.

But having attested to the value of physicians in any delivery system, we must also recognize that they have done a poor job of integrating themselves into the new paradigm. While 90 percent of health system executives surveyed agree that placing physicians squarely at the center of a network is crucial to its success, they are having major difficulties in accomplishing integration (*Modern Healthcare* 1997c), as shown by Figure 5.1. By and large, the overwhelming stumbling block is the resistance of physicians to change their traditional economic relationships. We have already discussed at length the problem most doctors have with change. Since physicians occupy an indispensable function, they are frequently in a position to sink any proposal not to their liking. This "spoil sport" attitude, while it may have been tolerated in the operating room, cannot continue if the medical profession is to achieve its potential for success under managed care.

The void created by the failure of hospitals, via their entities' HSNs, to reclaim the dominant role in delivery of care persists to this day. Hospitals, as the most organized and well-funded components of the system, were uniquely suited to step in behind the collapse of President Clinton's health plan and take over American medicine. I believe it is obvious why they have been unable to do so. Fixated on a defunct business model, they can never hope to be the agile, flexible user and deliverer of resources that the future will require. Even though hospitals continue to appear to dominate the medical market, they are already in decline; recall the diagram of the product life cycle of hospitals and consider the forces of cultural lag.

But with each decline comes opportunity. Physicians seem to be not unlike a disorganized marching band before a game. They are trained, skilled, and have the right instruments, but are just milling about for lack of coordination and leadership. As a result, two huge opportunities present themselves. The first is the big chance physician executives have been waiting for to allow them to rise to the fore. Over the past ten years, there has been a remarkable upsurge in the number of physicians who have taken the initiative to acquire the competencies required to lead healthcare organizations. This is no mean feat, given the historic

Cultural Lag

Cultural lag is a term popular with historians and sociologists. It refers to the start or end of an era that has occurred in every sense—culturally, economically, socially—except chronologically. Thus, the "Roaring Twenties" really ended well before 1930, and the antiestablishment movement that would be labeled as the Sixties really began in the late 1950s. One needs to look beyond the superficial to understand trends in a deeper and more meaningful way.

reluctance of doctors to be anything more than small businessmen. As the survey quoted above points out, it is still a problem for most systems to reach down into the rank and file of practitioners for support. But the growing class of physician executives is well situated to provide valuable service to any and all of the participants in the new medical marketplace.

Second, there is momentum, rising out of the vacuum of product leadership, for a unique alliance between health plans and medical groups. I term this the physician-payor axis because I envision it as the axis around which the entire delivery system will someday rotate. We are moving from a triad, as exemplified in the traditional fee-for-service scenario, to a dyad (see Figure 5.1). The triad was based on the premise that the physician worked in the hospital and both would receive charges-based reimbursement from a third party, usually with no questions asked. The paradigm involves a far more equal relationship between the physician and payor, with the hospital removed from the core of the delivery system. It becomes one more vendor of services to the system.

Figure 5.1 The Transition from Triad to Dyad

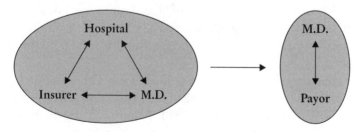

By changing the name of the insurer or third party to payor, I mean to suggest a new function, one that is far more proactive and interactive than collecting premiums and paying claims. The payor is acutely interested in all aspects of care, and has developed such tools as an extensive medical policy to match up against the procedures and services being delivered. This policy is designed to be an evidence-based resource for patient, physician, and payor to help with the complicated decisions surrounding cost-effective, outcomes-oriented medicine. Each member of the dyad, by virtue of the more egalitarian nature of the relationship, brings strengths and competencies to the other. Ideally it is a complementary interaction that is mutually reinforcing.

This design obviously goes well beyond a simple hub-and-spoke model that is the template for most HSNs and PHOs. Those organizations are predicated on static patterns of care, with the physical plant of the hospital and narrow geographical service area as the anchors. In a "virtual" world of constantly shifting needs and an escalating ability to access a host of resources configured to an individual case, such an approach is truly antiquated. Photographs of New York City from 1900 show the streets clogged with horses and carriages. Look closely, however, and you can see the occasional automobile. Their mere presence spelled the end of the horse-drawn era even as the number of horses in New York reached new highs.

The Imperatives of the Physician-Payor Axis

What I am proposing would seem anathema to many practitioners: stepping away from the long-held arrangements with hospitals to work directly with payors to develop networks for delivering care along radically different lines. There are several irresistible pressures that will continue to build and make this happen.

1. Employers are resistant to work with physicians

As much as physicians may resent the increasing influence of large employers in health decisions, employers dislike dealing with doctors. I am convinced most large companies, especially those without full-time medical directors, perceive physicians as the root cause of escalating healthcare costs.

This is not necessarily an unreasonable point of view. The variation in medical practice has been a recurrent theme of medical theorists for years (Greenfield et al. 1992; Gourfinkel et al. 1988). Admittedly, medicine is a mixture of art and science, so some variation in how a patient with a certain diagnosis is treated is probably good. In some circumstances, such as behavioral health, variation might even be encouraged and cherished. But when a patient presents with a diagnosis and receives radically different treatments, with no significant difference in outcomes, we have a problem. Typically this variation is accompanied by large discrepancies in costs. Rarely is medical evidence available to justify such variation.

The surprise for most physicians and hospitals is that large companies know about these costs and outcomes in much greater detail than they do. GM is the largest private purchaser of healthcare in the world and has amassed an impressive database on its employees' claims. When some of this information, such as in Figure 5.2, is presented to a medical audience, the reaction is often one of shock: first, because of what the figures say, and second, because someone who is not in medicine (an auto company of all things!) possesses such detailed knowledge of what doctors do. Between the data reflected in Figure 5.2, the stiff resistance of the AMA to any new healthcare initiative, and the unremitting increases in costs and volumes of services over the past 50 years, corporations have lost faith in physicians' ability or desire to address these issues effectively. In addition, they tend to feel more comfortable with insurers. Insurers and businesses have worked together for decades and speak the same language. If PSNs want to access employers, the most efficient route will be through, and with, payors.

Figure 5.2   Example of the Health Data Collected by Employers: GM Enrollees Filling Beta Blocker Scripts Post-MI, by Community

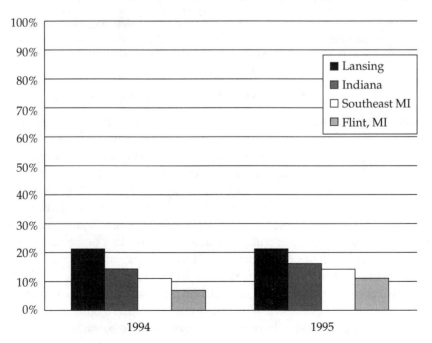

2. Payors have the necessary competencies

Doctors are smart people and are steeped in medical culture. This does not mean they understand insurance functions, or are capable of constructing proper risk arrangements, writing contracts, designing benefits, etc. This is truly the province of the insurer. Further, a long-term relationship should be the goal of any PSN-payor-employer venture. To support medical activities over the long haul demands a complex infrastructure that is constantly nourished, reworked, and modified. Can a small PSN or HSN HMO do this? For 20,000–50,000 lives, possibly. But for the kind of volume represented by a regional network, say 200,000 lives—definitely not. Recall the earlier discussions of the integrated delivery system (IDS). Too much energy needs to be devoted to its maintenance to allow an IDS to appropriately perform clinically. What is really needed is a "virtual" partner, one who can share information and provide support, but who does not demand resources to maintain a physical plant. The PSN must know its limitations and play to its strengths. Just as a payor should not practice medicine, a PSN should not dabble in insurance functions.

> **Case Study: Why Running an Insurance Company Is Not Something Just Any Idiot Can Do (Contrary to What Most Doctors Think)**
>
> Aetna U.S. Healthcare's value dropped 30 percent during 1997 as it suffered a major claims backup as a result of restructuring and its recent merger. Once the claims were cleared up, a higher-than-expected medical expense ratio was discovered, which had been masked by the mountain of claims. This in turn led to the product being underpriced, since the true medical cost trend had been obscured. Losses were in the tens of millions (*Wall Street Journal* 1997a).

3. Physicians need support to build a delivery platform

Coordinated care across a region for a large group of customers is new for physicians. The standard approach to practice-building for a medical group, or even a hospital, has been direct marketing and recruiting patients one by one. Managed care has redefined this process. A company with 500 employees will sign with a carrier and deliver all 500 on the effective date. For example, on January 1, the payor will gain a bolus of members that is then passed on to the providers. A physician may then see a significant increase in panel size in a matter of days or weeks. Conversely, if a payor loses a contract, that block of patients may suddenly leave a medical group's panel if it is not a provider for the payor to which the enrollees have migrated. The capability to deliver care in this new dynamic must be developed. The quickest and most effective manner of doing this is a partnership between the physician and payor.

> **A Few More Words on the IDS from Healthcare Futurist Jeff Goldsmith:**
>
> "Health care organizations cling to failed strategies: they marry their mistakes. The old industrial model of vertical integration doesn't work in industry anymore, so why are we using it in health care? Integrated delivery systems have discovered there are few or no buyers for many of their new products. Through mergers and acquisitions, these systems have accumulated both physical and human capital. Their theories about what would happen once they reached a certain mass or scale are not proving to be valid. Simply getting larger created all sorts of collateral problems, such as having 30,000 employees instead of 10,000 employees. The most important integration that needs to occur is integration people notice when they use the products or services" (*Medical Network Strategy Report* 1997).

4. The need to achieve improved outcomes propels payors and physicians to come together but pushes both away from the hospital

Outcomes measurement will be the mantra of managed care for the next ten years. It will probably take that long for everyone to get it right. HEDIS and the National Committee on Quality Assurance (NCQA) (and belatedly the Joint Commission on Accreditation of Healthcare Organizations [JCAHO]) have partially focused on outcomes but are still largely concerned with process. They will soon be eclipsed by the Foundation for Accountability (FAACT), a joint project among employers, unions, consumer groups, and health plans. FAACT's objectives are almost entirely outcomes-based, which can be seen, for example, by examining the parameters to be measured for assessing the quality of breast cancer care (see Table 5.2). It can be readily appreciated that this information is substantially different from simply reporting rates of mammograms and Pap smears. Not only does it require a different data collection process (meaning major information systems rework), but it entails looking at the world differently. That the patient went home from the hospital alive and ambulatory is not a sufficient end point. How is she at six months: at work? functioning independently? requiring certain levels of chronic care?

This type of longitudinal analysis, focused on outcomes that matter to individuals as well as employers (and society as a whole), cannot be effectively done by independent medical groups. Such studies are in effect population-based (and must be to have statistical validity and to be generalized to the public) and are a competency of the payor. The result is a natural alliance between the PSN and payor in this effort. At the same time, it moves the PSN-payor dyad away from the hospital

Table 5.2 Foundation for Accountability (FAACT) — Breast Cancer: Summary of Measures and Methodology

Measure	Performance Value	Instrument/Data Source
	Steps to Good Care	
Mammography	*Proportion* of women age 52–69 who have had a mammogram within a two-year period	Doctor's billing or claims records (NCQA's HEDIS 3.0 Breast Cancer Screening measure used)
Early stage detection	*Proportion* of patients whose breast cancer was detected at Stage 0 or Stage I	Patient records from cancer registry
Information about radiation treatment options	*Proportion* of Stage I and Stage II patients who indicate that they had adequate information about their radiation treatment options before deciding about surgical treatment	One question in patient satisfaction survey completed three to six months after diagnosis
Breast conserving surgery	*Proportion* of Stage I and Stage II patients who undergo breast conserving surgery	Patient records from cancer registry or claims records
Radiation therapy following breast conserving surgery	*Proportion* of breast conserving surgery patients who receive radiation treatment after breast conserving surgery	Patient records from cancer registry or claims records
	Experience and Satisfaction	
Patient satisfaction with care	*Mean* score for patients' level of satisfaction with breast cancer care, including technical quality, inter-personal and communication skills of their cancer doctor, involvement in treatment decisions, and timeliness of information and services	Thirty-two-item questionnaire patient survey completed three to six months after diagnosis
	Results	
Experience of disease	*Mean* score for patients on CARES-SF survey, which assesses patients' quality of life and experience in living with breast cancer	Fifty-nine-item CARES-SF patient survey compelted 12 to 15 months after diagnosis
Five-year disease-free survival (cancer treatment center measure)	*Probability* of disease-free survival for a group of patients, Stages I–IV, who were diagnosed during prior five years	Patient records from cancer registry

Source: The Foundation for Accountability, October 1997.

because the inpatient component becomes reduced to one of a series of care episodes. The value of the hospital piece becomes less than it was under the old fee-for-service approach. Many admissions and procedures do little to improve outcomes. Yet this inpatient activity is the heart of the hospital industry. Regardless of what hospital systems may say, an overriding part of their energy is spent filling beds (*Modern Healthcare* 1997b). Whenever this conflicts with, or does not directly promote, improved outcomes, hospitals diverge from the direction that the dyad needs to follow.

Physicians need tools to be successful in obtaining good outcomes. Development of such tools will eventually cost millions of dollars. Such expenditures are feasible for payors but are unlikely for more than a handful of well-heeled hospital systems. Because of their close links with industry, payors are also better suited to learn from the successful efforts of companies that have improved quality and outcomes.

An interesting example of improving outcomes industry involved Deere and Company. Productivity and quality of the product (i.e., the outcome) were in trouble. One problem was the multitude of training and repair manuals that were floating around. Too many were out of date and too much variation existed in training and work effort. Deere threw out every paper manual and put all relevant information on computers scattered throughout the plants. This virtual manual system could then be updated instantly and frequently. For the first time, all workers had access to the latest information, which was uniform across the company. A further interesting touch: none of it could be printed out, so the temptation to print a few key pages and stick them in a pocket or locker (where they might become outdated) was eliminated. It was a nice example of thinking outside the box.

5. The rate of new product development is increasing rapidly

Customization is hitting managed care hard. As we move into the adolescence of managed care, consumers are demanding many different products than a few years ago. Antimanaged care legislation is driving some of this change as well as health plans' struggle to remove some of the unpopular restrictions that have not been shown to decrease utilization or increase value. Open access is the new wave, with plans offering various methods of going directly to a specialist without passing through a gatekeeper (Humana, Inc., 1997; *Wall Street Journal* 1997c). Obviously physicians will be greatly affected by such products, not only because they affect their practices, but also because the design of these products will dictate care patterns for the future. It is a natural confluence for PSNs and payors to be intimately involved in this process together. To overcome the reluctance of payors to share decision making with physicians, PSNs need to be ready to accept risk, align financial incentives, and demonstrate their commitment (*Modern Healthcare* 1997a).

PSN-Payor Network Models

As with any network formation activity, a host of models are possible. Payors are aggressively developing new structures in the quest to find the ideal, which would accomplish several purposes. Consider the following examples or templates.

Integrated Joint Venture Model

The next step beyond a traditional independent practice association (IPA) model, a joint venture, involves the payor and medical group sharing ownership and integrating key services. A complicated contractual relationship also may result, with physicians and the payor owning the joint venture but the same physicians becoming contracted providers of the venture at the same time. Contracts would be developed with the various ancillary providers, including hospitals. Corporate profits would be driven by the ability of the payor to move greater market share into the sphere of the joint venture. This would work best if the payor commands a significant market share in the region. It is possible that the joint venture would have multipayor capabilities, but some conflict would likely result with the payor-owner. Because the partnering physicians are owners, they play a major role in governance, raising the level of autonomy enjoyed by the physicians who practice within it (see the next section for a more detailed discussion of autonomy issues). Because the hospital link is bypassed, there is more freedom in designing care patterns that are efficient.

Some negatives of this model affect both partners. Each would have some diminution of control and each would have to share profits. The reputation of the group as well as the health plan would affect the success of the venture in the market. The group would experience greater outside surveillance of its delivery of care, since there is an equity relationship with the payor. The tensions between specialists and primary care physicians might be amplified with such a close tie to a payor, involving direct governance. This would be an opportunity for a strong physician executive to exert leadership and deal with these conflicts proactively.

One caveat would be to consider nonexclusive arrangements in both directions: that is, both payor and provider can contract with outsiders if there is a compelling business reason to do so. This may help prevent excessive costs from being institutionalized by the artificial need to work within the joint venture alone.

Ownership Model

This model takes the joint venture to the extreme by placing all the physicians in the payor's direct employment. Most frequently this is done by direct purchase of smaller networks or large group practices. The payor controls all managed care responsibilities. The group is "captive." This means steady income to the physicians but transfers oversight to an external agent.

This is the least successful model. The experience of staff model HMOs, analogous to this model, have been disappointing in the last 20 years. Managing salaried physicians is a problem in terms of productivity and adherence to protocols, referral patterns, etc. This may seem to be a dichotomy since the physicians would appear to be under the greatest amount of control. But the highly specialized work physicians do and the difficulty in motivating people who are immune to many of the standard motivational tools (salary, incentives, threat of dismissal, etc.) makes this a challenging task. As many medical directors lament, managing physicians is like herding cats. Managing staff physicians, who often have their employers over a barrel in that it is almost impossible to replace them in less than several months, is even more exasperating. Added to this is periodic tension between salaried and consultant physicians, often involving money and volume of patients.

This may be a way to prepare the path to moving to a joint venture or other less controlled structure. It is instructive, though, to see the lack of return on investment that many purchasers of practices have seen.

Multipayor Model

The payor is one of several investors in a large network that also contracts with other payors. The physicians within and without the group are also investors, resulting in a better alignment of incentives. The lethargy that plagues the "owned" physicians discussed above is replaced by a more entrepreneurial spirit that allows for better access, higher quality goals, etc. Delegation of managed care functions to the physicians is key. The physician network provides the bulk of these activities (such as credentialing, utilization management, and case management,), leading to consistency across all products and books of business, as well as savings.

This framework is positive for employers because it can offer employees several payors at once and avoid the sudden, gut-wrenching shifts of large blocks of members that can happen as coverage changes.

Even though several payors are offered, there is standardization across the PSN. This option is also positive for the group since administrative savings accrue by not having to do the same tasks for different payors. By taking on as much delegated activity as it can handle, the group increases its autonomy and control of important functions. Last, this is positive for payors. As the group's efficiency increases, it is able to accept a lower capitation or other reimbursement. This allows the payor to directly benefit, along with the PSN, in the increased efficiency of the delivery of care. It also means the entity is well positioned to take advantage of one of the most important trends in managed care for the near term, namely accepting Medicare and Medicaid risk contracts. This is already a major revenue generator for many plans and physicians and will only become more valuable as states continue to move their Medicaid populations into managed care and as the percentage of retirees in Medicare HMOs increases.

This strategy is risky when multiple payors are roughly equal in the marketplace in terms of share, diluting the ability of the PSN to promote brand identity. As demonstrated by the current initiative in California to link medical groups and plans more closely in the public's mind, the necessity of raising the profile of the PSN is becoming more apparent. Part of this will involve creating brand identity as companies have done in other industries. We need only to look at the Permanente group to see the power of brand identity. PSNs will need to heighten awareness of this attribute, which may be affected by the number of payors who become part of the multipayor model.

At the same time, this negative is muted somewhat by the cushion the PSN enjoys because of the multiplicity of participating payors. The PSN, like any provider group, does not own the lives it serves. This is a difficult concept for physicians to accept, but it is true. It is further proof of the value of linking the physician and payor pieces to draw on the competencies of each, if only to ensure that the physicians are able to play on a level field without misunderstanding key concepts. The payors are able to move the lives they control from one provider to another, which is less of an issue under this model. It results in shifting a certain amount of leverage back to the PSN, restoring some of the all-important autonomy that physicians are so concerned about. Ideally the PSN and payor will find this relationship satisfying to the point that such movements are rare. As we move into more mature managed care, I think the radical shifts of members year to year—as employers and payors hunted down the very last cent of savings to be wrung from one group or another—are coming to an end. The emphasis on quality and customer service, which is incompatible with this approach, is precluding these swings of membership.

As a consequence, this model really works best in markets where the network has market share dominance. This will mean that it may be problematic in areas of fierce competition, especially in limited geographic areas. Yet as the consolidation of payors and providers continues, this may fade as an issue. The source of capital and the incentive to accept more lives from higher paying payors—both of which can affect the independence of the PSN and damage relationships with other, less well-funded payors—needs to be considered carefully in such high-competition service areas.

No model is perfect. The obligation really rests with the PSN and the physician members to assess local conditions to most accurately predict success. In general, a joint venture may have the best chance of doing well in most markets, especially when acquisition costs are high and there is a group of dominant payors. Ownership will always be risky if the plan is not a heavy player with deep pockets and a lion's share of the market. Remember: *Not all payors are alike.*

That payors differ as much as medical groups should be well known. There is a variety of strategic purposes behind the different forms of PSN-payor models. We sometimes tend to look at healthcare in homogeneous tones: all providers want to be high quality; all payors want to deliver strong products at the lowest price. Such uniformity does not exist in other markets. There is a top-of-the-line automobile, an economy version, a mid-range model, etc. We are moving into an era when providers and payors will begin to differentiate themselves more completely than in the past. In the book *The Discipline of Market Leaders*, Treacy and Wiersma (1995) speak of three types of leadership in modern markets. They are outlined in Table 5.4. Consider the description of each type and the company that uses it as its strategic purpose. Hopefully it will be evident how each of these companies exemplifies this direction. Wal-Mart is a combination of price, quality, and convenience. Toyota produces an outstanding product that often commands a premium price. Nordstrom will do whatever is necessary to please an individual customer, including giving extraordinary personal service that may well cost more than the item purchased.

One of the basic points of the theory of market discipline is that it creates a value proposition: an implicit promise to deliver the particular value the customer desires. This value proposition is similar for all enterprises that embrace it, across various industries. That is, whether a company is in auto manufacturing, electronics, food services, or healthcare, if it has chosen to pursue a certain market discipline, its value discipline (the

Table 5.3 Three Types of Leadership in Modern Markets

Leadership Discipline	Characteristics (Key Proposition to Customers)	Example
Operational Excellence	Offers low price and hassle-free service; are not primarily product or service innovators; do not seek deep, one-on-one relationships with customers	Wal-Mart: no frills approach to mass marketing
Product Leadership	Create and offer the best product, pushing performance limits through continuous innovation	Toyota: excellence of product often commands a premium price
Customer Intimacy	Focuses on what particular customer wants; cultivates relationships; understands customer and seeks to satisfy unique needs	Nordstrom: will consistently go the extra mile for its selectively chosen customers

Source: Michael Treacy, Fred Wiersma. *The Discipline of Market Leaders.* Reading, MA: Addison-Wesley Publishing Company, 1995, p. xiii.

manner in which operating models and value propositions are combined) will be similar to others regardless of what it is actually producing. It becomes industry-independent.

This idea is important to drive home the point that we are on the threshold of a similar breakout of health plans and, ultimately, medical groups. Many health plans will link with PSNs and will choose the type of discipline they will use to succeed. Some will focus on being the lower cost solution, appealing perhaps to small employers on tight budgets. Some will offer highly developed products, rich with sophisticated components such as advanced disease state management, health risk assessments, multiple case management options, etc. Others will be able to address specialized needs such as home care that includes housekeeping, transportation, and other services that are usually not thought of as being medically related, yet are necessary to achieve satisfactory outcomes for complicated cases that do not fit a routine pattern.

This breakout will present both challenges and opportunities for the PSN. Its solution to this spectrum of niche payors may be to create a "portfolio" of them in order to deliver a wide range of options to potential members as it seeks to build market share. By allowing the payors to develop and support their separate core competencies, a PSN can concentrate on the actual delivery of medical care (which is *its* core competency). The interaction between the payor and the PSN becomes complementary, even symbiotic. And being symbiotic, it avoids duplication of effort and achieves maximum efficiency and effectiveness.

The Future Is Now

As the relationship between the deliverer (the PSN) and the payor matures, the PSN-payor axis will become mutually reinforcing. The strengths of each partner will be bolstered by not having to divert resources outside its core competency. The PSN, and the individual physician member, may be concerned that this close tie may serve to diminish the profile of the provider with the public, to subsume the physician piece within the dyad. I believe the reverse will occur, and that, in fact, the visibility of the PSN will be much greater under this model than in the current situation. This will be a gigantic opportunity for physician executives to lead the entire medical community into an entirely new medical system.

With the PSN-payor axis as the core of the medical delivery system, the vendors of ancillary services (hospitals, outpatient clinics, home health agencies, etc.) will step into a secondary role. They will essentially be on a shelf, to be chosen by the provider as needed. The front-line contact for the vast majority of Americans will be the PSN. On the doors of the PSN may be the name of the principal payor with which the PSN has joined. If the PSN has elected the portfolio approach, several names will be there. More than ever, people will be aware of the unique identities of the organizations delivering and supporting their medical care. As employers try to reduce their employee offerings, they will need to know details of the PSN performance separate from that of the health plans. Medical groups will find themselves directly scrutinized by both patients and employers, as well as payors and the government.

This identification has already begun in California, as one might expect from the cradle of the HMO movement. In 1997, for the first time, the Pacific Business Group on Health (PBGH), an influential employer group that has long rated health plans, began issuing report cards on large medical groups (*San Francisco Chronicle* 1997). It surveyed 25,000 patients of 49 Northern California medical groups to determine satisfaction, preventive care, access, etc. Admittedly a crude first pass, it is nevertheless a significant shift in how we have usually looked at healthcare. Until now, the onus has fallen almost entirely on the health plan and the hospital. NCQA and JCAHO only indirectly reflected what went on in the physician's office. FAACT is heading in that direction, but it is years away. Quality has always been defined independently by each physician in the fee-for-service milieu. As the PBGH approach spreads and becomes more refined, this will change. Choosing a medical delivery system—not just a doctor—will involve evaluating both health plan and

medical group/PSN. The importance of the PSN will rise as a consequence, reinforcing the complementary nature of the PSN-payor axis.

Autonomy and Ethics

Implementation of this axis will not be as daunting as it may appear.
At this stage in the evolution of managed care, both payors and PSNs
have certain responsibilities to make the decision to move forward. On
balance, the ball is probably slightly more in the physicians' court. The
current withering attacks on managed care continue unabated. Because
the Clinton health plan was shot down as too much government interfer-
ence, the route of government involvement in healthcare operations has
increased dramatically. Much of it has been led, ironically, by the same
coalition that destroyed the administration's plan: doctors, consumer
groups, state legislators. It is both schizophrenic and hypocritical. As an
outcome of the slowing of the growth and development of managed care
(*Wall Street Journal* 1997b), the impetus needs to shift to the PSN side.
Hopefully, as PSNs continue to form and mature, they will soon pick up
the slack and move forward to build these alliances.

Once the decision is made to proceed, the ideas will automatically fall
into place on how to establish an effective partnership. Prime among these
is the issue of autonomy. Long a sensitive topic for doctors, this issue
must be reconciled within the new operating framework. I am optimistic.
I see the PSN-payor link as giving a new birth to physician autonomy.
It will not be the wide-open, no-restrictions system of the fee-for-
service past. That was not good for anyone—patients, insurers, society,
even physicians. The power to make decisions about other people's
lives with other people's money in a vacuum with no oversight was
not healthy. Autonomy means self-direction and moral independence,
but also implies a measure of oversight and certainly a large degree
of accountability. As PSNs assume responsibility for the clinical end
of care, within the context of a payor partnership and recognizing the
obligation to achieve positive outcomes, the autonomy of the practitioner
will be extensive. It will be a more satisfying style of practice than when
the doctor was hobbled by a referral process, audited by claims, etc.
These punitive tactics are part of a system predicated on an adversarial
arrangement between doctor and payor, with each mistrusting the other.
Neither understands the other's objectives or respects the other's tasks.
Each impinges on the other's turf, making conflict inevitable. Autonomy
is compromised, and neither party is happy. It is a very paternal approach
to what should be a sophisticated interaction.

By devolving accountability and responsibility on each, pulling back to attend to competencies only, and trusting the other to work toward a mutually beneficial goal, we move beyond this scenario. The irony is that this direction is so basic, even simple. Yet as former President Ronald Reagan said, "The right things to do are often simple, they're just not easy."

As we develop this new structure both to deliver better care (i.e., care that improves the health status of Americans) and to strengthen physician autonomy, the PSN-payor alliance will permit physicians to perform an important ethical obligation. Medical professionals have always recognized their ethical duty to individual patients. This approach should not be changed in the future. But there is an ethical responsibility to society as well. As the American College of Obstetricians and Gynecologists states in its Code of Professional Ethics: "The [physician] should support and participate in those health care programs, practices and activities that contribute positively, in a meaningful and cost-effective way, to the welfare of individual patients, the health care system, or the public good" (1997). Perhaps for the first time ever, the broad majority of physicians will be involved constructively in such efforts, realizing their ethical responsibility to the nation as a whole.

References

American College of Obstetricians and Gynecologists. 1997. *Code of Professional Ethics.*

Gourfinkel, S. A., G. F. Riley, and V. G. Iannachionne. 1988. "High-Cost Users of Medical Care." *Health Care Financing Review* 9 (4): 41–52.

Greenfield, S., E. C. Nelson, M. Zubkoft, et al. 1992. "Variations in Resource Utilization among Medical Specialties and System of Care: Results from the Medical Outcomes Studies." *Journal of the American Medical Association* 267: 1623–30.

Humana Inc. 1997. "Humana Gold Plus Plan: How to Get Better Coverage Than with Medicare Alone."

Medical Network Strategy Report. 1997. "IDS Survival Strategies." 6 (7): 3–8.

Modern Healthcare. 1997a. 1 September: 68.

———. 1997b. 22 September: 60.

———. 1997c. "The Reluctant Doctor." 1 September: 66.

San Francisco Chronicle. 1997. "Pick a Health Team, Not Just a Doc." 22 September: B1-B5.

Treacy, M., and F. Wiersma. 1995. *The Discipline of Market Leaders.* Reading, MA: Addison-Wesley Publishing Company.

Wall Street Journal. 1997a. 1 October: B-13.

———. 1997b. "Quality of HMOs in U.S. Varies Widely, Report by Accreditation Group Finds." 2 October: B6.

———. 1997c. "New Medicare Rules Offer More Options—And Worries." August: B1.

6

BEYOND MANAGED CARE

"The result of movement toward integrated delivery will be that we in Catholic health care become responsible for people, not property. Consider for a moment the awesome responsibility and potential for ministry that comes from being accountable not just for the provision of service but for the health status of defined communities. What opportunities for wellness, prevention, wholeness and quality of life!"
                                        —Mary Kathryn Grant, Holy Cross Health System, 1994

PARTICULARLY enjoy the above quotation because I can feel the enthusiasm and excitement that Ms. Grant is feeling. What she is really referring to is the new thinking that is the most important benefit healthcare and physician executives can derive from the entire managed care movement. As she describes the path she wishes her organization to follow, she is able to adapt it to the mission of the Catholic health systems. This mission is not substantially different from that of any medical delivery system that understands the new paradigm of focusing on health status versus an episode of illness. I am always distressed when I hear colleagues say they would not encourage their children to choose medicine as a career. Their "golden era," if it ever existed, may be drawing to a close, but we stand on the threshold of the greatest opportunity ever to change medical care fundamentally for the better. I have sought throughout this book to convey some sense of why this is true and how networks will be an integral part of this transformation.

Because networks are a facilitator of medical care delivery, they will necessarily mirror the evolution of heathcare and, indeed, will be at the heart of any significant change. Based on the discussions, case studies, and analyses presented, it is hard to picture any meaningful or effective reorientation of care patterns that does not address the network issue. Two caveats are worth mentioning at this juncture. First, we must be careful not to mistake the means for the end. Networks are a facilitator. They are a tool to allow us to get the job of delivering the kinds of outcomes FAACT and other sophisticated oversight bodies will be expecting. The creation of the network itself must never be mistaken for the completion of the task. It is revealing to study networks formed in the heat of the healthcare battle of the mid-1990s that have gone exactly nowhere.

A Brief Case Study: The Network That Didn't

Northwestern University Medical Center in Chicago formed a much-ballyhooed network with north suburban Evanston Hospital in 1992. The match seemed to be ideal: Northwestern is a tertiary care center located in a fashionable section of downtown Chicago, and Evanston is in a well-to-do suburb (where many of the executives who work near Northwestern live, providing a certain symmetry). It was anticipated that significant patient volumes would result, with big-dollar managed care contracts bringing in thousands of lives. In late 1997, the two hospitals threw in the towel on their network after not a single "life" had been accrued as a result of the network. They will now reconfigure and try to jump-start the alliance under a different name and a new direction (*Modern Healthcare* 1997).

Hence, network formation is the process, not the engine. Without a clear, reality-based strategy for delivering a truly new way of providing medical care, the end result is likely to resemble that of Northwestern University Medical Center in Chicago.

Second, since the purpose of networks is to redirect care, and since networks are a tool, we should not fool ourselves into believing that they are in any sense a permanent structure. One of the (many) Achilles' heels of the hospital industry is the misconception that hospitals are eternal, that what was built on this site 60 years ago must, at all costs, continue on forever. Long after the economic and public value of many hospitals have vanished, boards of trustees and communities cling to their dinosaurean institutions. Meanwhile these institutions are left in the dust by fleeter competitors. The irony is that often such denial ends up hurting the people who are supposed to be served by preventing them from benefiting from more efficient and medically effective care. Likewise, we must acknowledge that as we progress along the evolutionary ladder of managed care and its successors, there will come a time when this model is no longer workable. We must be ready at that time to move off in a new and more technologically advanced direction as circumstances dictate. The danger is to become victims of "cultural lag" as discussed in Chapter 5.

What will happen to managed care? If there is any validity to the paragraph above, then the corollary is that managed care itself is a temporary phenomenon. This does not mean that the ostrich-like leaders of organized medicine and some state legislatures are correct, that managed care will collapse of its own steam and we will roll back to the fee-for-service structure of the past. Rather, this means that managed care is one stage on the timeline of medicine, a timeline that has been moving forward for decades. The distinguishing feature of the past few years is that the shifts and redirections have been fast and furious compared to the relatively indolent change of the previous 50 years. (Of course, the change of those decades appears incredibly swift compared to the first century and a half of American medicine. All things are relative.) What we will see in the next decade, if not sooner, is the emergence of the next level of managed care. Since the turn of the century, we have gone from medicine as a cottage industry, based largely on barter, to the complex beast it is today.

The next level will address the contradictions we have not been able to resolve to date. Medical care is more available today than ever, yet enormous access problems exist. Technology has brought us to the brink of manipulating and treating everything down to the level of individual amino acids. Meanwhile, children are still not immunized against the most basic infectious diseases. We have perfected a host of surgical techniques, but we are still unable to demonstrate that they make a difference in people's overall health. We are superb at treating individuals but lack the capacity to make dramatic headway in improving the health status of the nation as a whole. While costs continue to escalate, more people than ever have insurance and, ironically, more people than ever are uninsured. Then there is the question of why we should even need insurance to cover what is a basic service; no one has food insurance.

What the next stage of managed care will do is focus on these and other value-related issues. We reap undeniable benefits from our medical care system, but do we receive *value*? The answer for most people is no, and that will be the challenge for the next few years. The ability to deliver and then to monitor outcomes will be the nut to crack.

The Next Important Breakthrough

Managed care was a critical breakthrough. It made us think about questions that had not seemed important in the past. In the 1980s, who cared about costs? Not the lay public, that's for sure. Only when the cost of our profligate system reached a critical mass did we suddenly realize there was a problem. Today many still do not accept that there is a problem, although they are generally people who have access to health insurance at a reasonable cost and for whom delivery issues are just not on the radar.

The next big movement will be to hone in on outcomes and measurement. This will go hand-in-hand with accountability, which is where networks will be an indispensable tool. As FAACT and others work to make outcomes the mantra of the next wave, the PSN-payor axis will find itself coming into its own (see Chapter 5). Centered as it is around accountability and responsibility, it will be a natural starting point for developing the protocols to produce and collect this data. The first step is to center the PSN-payor partnership around best practices (i.e., critical pathways, specifications of acceptable care, or whatever appellation one chooses to use). The standardization of care, anchored upon medical evidence, is the objective. The ability to benchmark and compare across plans and regions has of yet eluded us. This will be a necessary development in the near future to allow us to determine if in fact our interventions are making any difference. As always, the emphasis has to be on value: the best outcomes at an acceptable cost. However, the issue of cost will become secondary as consumers come to believe that (for the first time ever) they are receiving care that truly is effective for their healthcare dollar.

With the virtual integration of the PSN and payor systems, data collection will be less of an obstacle than it currently is. Comprehensive profiles of the community, of the physician, and of the plan members will be essential building blocks of the new care patterns, and will have a multitude of secondary benefits. For the first time, we will know the impact of these new networks and will be able to modify them as necessary. All of this experience will feed into the refinement of the new managed care paradigm and give it a different face from the one we now know. This knowledge of whether people are actually better off with the medical care they receive would then lead us to the next level of sophistication, the healthcare coalition.

The Healthcare Coalition

Formed of PSNs, payors, and possibly some employers, such coalitions would cross a variety of PSN-payor organizations and be devoted to improving the health of the population of a region. These will not be a rehash of the entities proposed under President Clinton's plan to manage competition and dole out federal moneys. Rather, they would be almost spontaneously forming in response to the information being gathered on what works and what does not. Being able to correlate the success of an intervention with its cost, time, and resources required will be a powerful motivator for the interested parties to work in concert to implement the interventions that prove themselves. Those treatments that do not justify themselves will be discarded or relegated to an "alternative medicine" category that would be accessible to customers, but at their own cost and risk. This process will be sped along by the further consolidation of the market on the payor side. As fewer companies exist, they will have a larger market share and their market power will enable them to drive down operating costs and increase standardization.

The upshot will be increased profits for all participants. (This includes practitioners. There is no reason to believe any of these changes will put pressure on their incomes any more than what has already occurred. Even as managed care accounted for ever-increasing percentages of total patient census, most specialties have seen net income increases ahead of inflation for the past five years.) Indeed, even patients and employers will benefit economically from this shift. Effective care will be less wasteful care, and as the burden of health costs stabilizes or even declines, the paying public will notice. A secondary benefit also may be a move away from the need to underwrite extensively; with improved health status, the risk to insurers decreases. The lowered costs should be translated into lowered premiums (which may also help in some way address the problem of access to affordable insurance).

What does this mean for individual physicians? As they regain control of the core processes of healthcare delivery, autonomy will increase, as we have shown. I believe that satisfaction will increase as well. Doctors want to do the right things for their patients. Once they can be presented with the evidence of the positive outcomes of the approaches to care being outlined, they eventually will accept and support them. A period of acclimation is required. After all, it took several years for most physicians to understand that Medicare was not a Soviet plot. Physicians will need to come to grips with the new philosophy of the next stage of managed care; this will be a tall order admittedly, since many have not yet come to terms with the present incarnation of managed care.

The demise of micromanagement, inherent in the movement to the next level, may help. Physicians rightly chafe under the restrictions, many of them punitive, of managed care. These rules were never intended to be so negative. I see them as a reflection of the lack of sophistication of the original designers of the HMO model. This is not a criticism as much as a recognition that in the genesis of any new system, particularly one so complex as medical care, refinement of the processes will only come with time and learning. We have seen the mixed results of looking over the shoulder of the practitioner, and they are not impressive. The new model will have incorporated those lessons and moved beyond such inefficiencies. Far more important is getting physicians to embrace the new philosophy and build a trend in that direction. As stated earlier, we are excellent at treating the individual patient but poor at treating the population. The task for the physician, in order to be free to include some variation in his or her practice to suit the individual, is to work at implementing the systems to serve the population. With the acceptance of responsibility and accountability, the necessity to control the care obsessively at a microscopic level becomes even less appropriate.

This ultimately will lead to yet another iteration of the value equation and value diagram. Recall the discussion of value in Chapter 3. This was based on the current understanding of what the players in the healthcare arena want now and will want in the future. In the near future, the issue will be how to lure, not drive, potential members into new care delivery structures. This will mean approaching the benefits and services these members derive from membership in a new light. It will mean making the benefits more attractive and useful (i.e., increasing the value of the benefits) as well as creating a new setting in which those benefits will be seen. As shown in Figure 6.1, the interaction between the value components will become even more complex, fascinating, and important.

Of course, success will have its own ramifications. As the health status of people begins to improve, this alone will start to redefine the patterns of care. While practices as micromanagement will go away, others will become more prominent. For example, PSNs will have less tolerance for physicians who are excessive utilizers when high volumes of procedures

Figure 6.1 Future Concepts of Value and Its Components

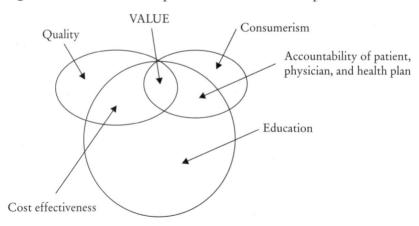

are no longer justifiable based on the severity index of the population. This will be the result of trend analyses that give a higher level view of care being delivered, but that are more relevant to a large cohort of patients: just the kind of data that employers, and indeed the healthcare coalition charged with caring for a group versus a series of individuals, will find terribly important to their decision making.

It also means that as new trends become clear, problems that are unknown to us today will come to the fore and demand attention. One lesson from the past five years has been that we can often see where we want to go but cannot get there until more pressing needs are addressed. This in turn may frequently lead us to issues that are not apparent until we take a certain pathway to reach a distant goal. This will be an ever more common situation. In 1990, healthcare leaders knew we had to do something radical to reorient the medical care delivery pattern, but the objectives of outcomes and measurement were not yet understood.

Despite the dire forecasts of the opponents of change, the increase in PSN-payor cooperation will not mean the end of specialists. Quite the contrary: the advent of effective PSNs, working in tandem with payors in the framework we have discussed, will mean the survival of many specialties that would otherwise be seriously threatened if nothing is done. Take, for example, infertility treatment. The recent advances that are the grist of Sunday newspaper supplements are incredibly expensive, as most people know. Under the traditional system, the number of patients who can afford these treatments is rapidly declining because of basic economics. Left unchanged, only the very rich would be able to avail themselves of the latest and most effective reproductive technologies. This in turn would mean a markedly reduced number of infertility providers. With infertility incorporated into most managed care plans, and with the PSN acting as an expert intermediary between patient, payor, and specialist (who may or may not belong to the PSN), the future for this specialty will be much more secure (Cohen 1996).

Value, Quality, and Results

The touchstone for the future is value. This concept has been conspicuously absent in healthcare. Recall the value equation from Chapter 3. This is really what everyone is after. Boiling down the demands of consumers, employers, the government, and even physicians themselves, it basically amounts to receiving a product or service that is considered of value with respect to the resources expended. Those who are not happy with medical costs feel too much is spent for too little benefit. Those who provide medical care complain that they are doing the best they can and that this is what care costs. The framework that can reconcile these conflicting views will hold the magic bullet to resolving many of our conflicts about healthcare.

Quality is inherent in value, but the reverse is not necessarily true. As those involved in redesigning the medical care system, our obligation is to make it true. High quality can no longer be seen as a differentiating factor, but simply as the "ticket for admission" that all must have in order to participate. Once admitted, the challenge will be to add that elusive component—value. This will be contingent on the kinds of outcomes that a network can demonstrate. These results must also be generated in a different context than we have done to date. Physicians and consumers are tired of punitive financial arrangements; they look bad, smell bad, and do not work (*Managed Care* 1997). They will hopefully disappear over the next two to three years as we become more comfortable with the idea of trusting providers to adhere to managed care philosophy, and as new tools are created to measure outcomes reliably and meaningfully. This will be a big step forward.

PSNs and payors also need to be willing to take the long view of profitability. We have all become too obsessed with health costs and personal incomes. Physicians scream if their reimbursement goes down; employers do the same if premiums go up. As the new alignment of physicians and payors takes shape, and hospitals and other ancillaries assume their new secondary, supporting roles, a transitional structure will necessarily come into being. During this time it is less important to realize maximum return on investment than to put in place a system that will dominate the medical delivery system for the future, and do so in a constructive manner.

Maintaining the momentum of change will be the responsibility of all involved. The time for active or passive obstructionism is past, and those who continue to practice it are already being marginalized. Full profit and return on investment will come soon enough as the fundamental realignment discussed occurs. The key is discipline and focus, and a faith in the choices made by those sincerely committed to a new and better way to care for our citizenry.

In the midst of the Civil War, President Lincoln was asked to raise the flag over a new fort and deliver a dedication speech. In characteristic fashion, his remarks were brief yet cogent. His entire address consisted of one sentence that speaks to us as we move forward in this effort:

"The part assigned to me is to raise the flag, which, if there be no fault in the machinery, I will do, and when up, it will be for the people to keep it up" (Sandburg 1954).

References

Cohen, A. W. 1997. "Managed Health Care's Approach to Infertility." *Contemporary OB/GYN* June: 93–107.

Managed Care. 1997. "Health Plan Fines Doctors for Extra Hospital Days." August: 12.

Medical Economics. 1997. "OB/GYN's Earnings: Overdue for an Increase." September: 40–48.

Modern Healthcare. 1997. 2 October: 33.

Sandburg, C. 1954. *Abraham Lincoln*. New York: Harcourt Brace, 405.

INDEX

ABOUT THE AUTHOR

Derek van Amerongen, M.D., M.S., currently serves as national medical director for Anthem Blue Cross and Blue Shield in Cincinnati. He trained in obstetrics and gynecology at the University of Chicago and is board certified in obstetrics and gynecology. His experience has included community and inner-city OB/GYN practice, as well as over six years on the faculty of the Johns Hopkins School of Medicine in Baltimore. He is the author of numerous research, professional, and management articles and lectures extensively on managed care and health policy topics. A passionate proponent of the healthcare evolution, Dr. van Amerongen holds an A.B. from Princeton University, an M.D. from Rush Medical College, and an M.S. from the University of Wisconsin–Madison. Dr. van Amerongen lives in Cincinnati with his wife and three children.